The Parents' Concise Guide to
Childhood Vaccinations

The Parents' Concise Guide to
Childhood
Vaccinations

Practical Medical and Natural Ways
to Protect Your Child

Lauren Feder, M.D.
Author of *Natural Baby and Childcare*

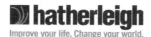

Improve your life. Change your world.

This book does not give legal or medical advice. Always consult your doctor, lawyer, and other professionals. Names of medications and products are typically followed by TM or ® symbols, but these symbols are not stated in this book.

The ideas and suggestions contained in this book are not intended as a substitute for consulting with a physician. All matters regarding your health require medical supervision.

Hatherleigh Press
5-22 46th Avenue, Suite 200
Long Island City, NY 11101
www.hatherleighpress.com

Library of Congress Cataloging-in-Publication Data
Feder, Lauren.
The parents' concise guide to childhood vaccinations : practical medical and natural ways to protect your child / Lauren Feder.
    p. cm.
ISBN 978-1-57826-251-9
1. Vaccination of children—Popular works. 2. Immunization of children—Popular works. 3. Vaccination of children—Complications—Risk factors. 4. Vaccines—Health aspects. I. Title.
RJ240.F43 2007
614.4'7083—dc22
                    2007022621

ISBN 978-1-57826-251-9

The Parents' Concise Guide to Childhood Vaccinations is available for bulk purchase, special promotions, and premiums. For information on reselling and special purchase opportunities, call 1-800-528-2550 and ask for the Special Sales Manager.

Interior design by Allison Furrer

Cover design by Allison Furrer

10 9 8 7 6 5 4 3 2 1

Printed in the United States

ACKNOWLEDGEMENTS

Many thanks to my editor, Andrea Au; the production team, including Deborah Miller, Allison Furrer, and Mary Jane DeFroscia; and the publicity/marketing team, including Kevin Moran and Mariel Dumas, for their dedication to the project. In addition, my gratitude extends to my agent, Jessica Faust.

To parents who I have worked with and share the common aim of raising happy and healthy children. To my family, friends, and my loving sons Étienne and Quentin, who inspired me to take this journey and supported me along the way.

And my deep appreciation to the philosopher Mervyn Brady and the students of the Academy of European Arts and Culture, whose infinite wisdom guides me along my journey.

Lauren Feder, M.D.
Los Angeles

To my mother, Ellie Davis,
who showed me the love of motherhood,
and my father, Dr. Robert J. Feder,
the love of medicine.

CONTENTS

The Vaccination Controversy

When I was growing up, going to the doctor for shots was a time honored tradition that we all accepted—like it or not! Even during my training as a resident at the hospital, I dutifully went for yearly physicals, which included an updating of the basic adult immunizations. Like my parents, I never questioned vaccinations and did not consider them anything but a normal part of routine prevention of illnesses. It wasn't until I was successfully treated for a thyroid condition with holistic medicine that I became interested in the complementary medical approach of using the body's natural defenses against disease as much as possible. In this view, vaccinations can interfere with the body's natural immunity and may themselves cause disease.

Vaccinations, which for decades had been hailed as one of the major achievements in public health, are no longer immune to controversy. In our grandparents' days, nearly all children had measles, mumps, and rubella. It's not uncommon to hear stories about chickenpox parties in our parents' days that flourished at the first sign of the rash when all the mothers would rush their children over to the infected child's house. Since the introduction of vaccines in the twentieth century, these common childhood diseases are no longer *common*. This would seem to be good news. But in recent years, professional journals and newspapers have reported with increasing frequency on vaccine injuries, mercury toxicity, and possible links between vaccinations and chronic diseases such as autism.

One of the first major health decisions facing new parents is whether or not to vaccinate. Many parents do not even realize there is a choice, as there has been the assumption that vaccinations are compulsory rather than voluntary for entry into school. Vaccinations are recommended by our healthcare system for every child. However, like any medication, vaccinations carry the risk of adverse effects and are not always 100 percent safe. Sometimes a child can experience a reaction after a shot—discomfort, allergic reactions, and even reports of death have occurred. Stories in the media about the link between autism and the measles, mumps, and rubella (MMR) shot are prevalent. As a result, a growing number of parents have begun to question the safety and effectiveness of vaccines. Nowadays, with the abundance of information available, parents are more informed about the health benefits and risks of vaccinations, pose more questions to their doctors, and are interested in taking some responsibility for their children's health and wellbeing. Some of my patients fully vaccinate to schedule, some not at all, and others vaccinate selectively.

The Current State of Our Children's Health

Medical advancements in the 1900s were impressive in their achievements: We are treating diseases with more sophisticated techniques, targeting illness with complex drugs and extensive therapeutic regimes. We understand the mechanics of the body better than at any time in history. But even as we are told we are healthier and living longer, more children every year are on daily medications for chronic conditions. In recent years, I have witnessed a dramatic increase in these sorts of conditions—children who suffer from repeated ear infections, severe asthma, allergies, or eczema, or even behavioral problems like Attention Deficit Hyperactivity Disorder (ADHD).

The explanations for the increase in chronic childhood illnesses are complex and often contradictory; the effects on children and families, however, are profound and evident. As a result, more parents every year confront the limits of conventional medicine in treating and addressing the causes of chronic illnesses like these.

Unfortunately, healthcare in the United States has a long way to go before it is satisfactory. According to an article in the *Journal of the American Medical Association* (Barbara Starfield, M.D., "Is U.S. Health Really the Best in the World?" JAMA. 2000; 284: 483–485) the United States ranked 12th out of a group of 13 countries when measured on health indicators such as low birth weight, infant mortality, and life expectancy. Our children, who represent the future generation, may be more at risk than we were. Many of our children, for instance, are ingesting more than safe amounts of fluoride from local water supplies, which damages tooth enamel, ligaments, muscles, and skin, and is associated with lower IQ levels, arthritis, and cancer. Mercury used in amalgam dental fillings is known to be toxic and may lead to damage to the brain, kidney, and immune system. Antibiotic overuse has caused antibiotic resistance, yeast overgrowth, and weakening of the immune system.

Nowadays, according to the American Obesity Association, 15 percent of children in the United States are obese, an increase of over 50 percent in children ages 6 to 11 since the 1960s. Most overweight adolescents grow up to become obese adults. This alarming rise in obesity has been blamed upon a number of societal causes, including our more sedentary lifestyle, high rates of television viewing (up to 30 hours a week), and the prevalence of fast food and junk food in school. In many elementary and high schools, it's not uncommon to find vending machines selling candy and soft drinks. With financial restrictions and cutbacks a reality at many schools, these machines have become a money-maker for the schools. To add to the obesity problem, physical education programs are among the first cut during school financial crises, and nationwide, children are increasingly deprived of exercise during school hours. Obesity brings with it a host of health problems: diabetes, heart disease, high blood pressure, and higher incidence of some cancers.

Also in recent years, the number of children diagnosed with learning and behavioral disorders, such as ADHD, dyslexia, auditory processing disorder, visual disability, Asperger's syndrome, and autism, has vastly increased. Learning disorders are known to affect 30 percent of children in the United States, according to the Scripps Howard News Service. Most research has been inconclusive as to the causes. Factors such as environmental pollution, poor nutrition, antibiotic overuse, and changes in family life have all fallen under suspicion as possible causes. However, many of the families in my office practice have witnessed adverse effects following vaccinations, and have come to blame vaccines for causing or contributing to these disorders.

With the health statistics stacked against our children in nearly every aspect of their lives, many parents and healthcare practitioners are interested in taking proactive measures to counter the odds. Doctors, even those who practice conventional medicine, are adopting a more holistic and preventive approach to healthcare. Most agree that maintaining and cultivating health demands more than simply prescribing medication. Wellbeing extends to the mind and spirit as well as the body and includes wholesome nutrition, exercise, healthy lifestyle, and harmony in relationships. During times of illness, many parents are turning to natural forms of medicine as a first line of defense, and employing conventional medication only when needed. Now many are also realizing that this attitude should also apply to vaccinations.

What's Right for My Child?

Whatever your decision regarding vaccinations, the goal is always the same: to raise happy and healthy children who are able to blossom and reach their potential in life. As a physician to many families, the most common question I hear from concerned parents is, "What should I do about the shots?" My response is that it depends upon your child's overall health status and risks for specific diseases or side effects, as well as upon your personal values.

As a physician trained in both standard and holistic medicine, I am privy to two ways of thinking about health. As an M.D., I am well aware that the standard of care is to vaccinate; as a holistic practitioner, I recognize that vaccinations can present short-term and sometimes long-term risks for both children and adults. Although the goals of conventional and holistic medicine are the same, the approaches can be vastly different, and the choices offered can be confusing and even frustrating for parents.

After careful consideration of the options, my husband and I decided not to vaccinate our children. In my office practice and in my lectures, however, I am careful to emphasize that our decision to not vaccinate was a personal family decision, and as a caretaker to many families, I do not impose this course of action on my patients. I recognize that vaccinations prevent many severe and life-threatening illnesses, and it would be naïve to trust that healthy lifestyles and natural parenting approaches are always going to provide us with adequate solutions. Although homeopaths have been treating infectious diseases successfully for several centuries, I would not hesitate to rely on medicine and technical advancements of the twenty-first century when needed. My book *Natural Baby and Childcare* gives more information about both natural and medical treatments for many of these illnesses.

The decision to vaccinate can be a confusing and difficult one for some families, as we all want to do what is right for our children. Some parents base their decision on statistics in books and on the Internet. From the Centers for Disease Control and Prevention (CDC) to the National Vaccine Information Center (NVIC), which was begun by parents whose children were injured following vaccinations, the data can vary. Some people base their decision on personal experience; they know someone who is crippled with polio, or they suffered an adverse side effect from a vaccine.

Whatever your decisions, I strongly support a "pro-informed-choice" attitude—one that encourages you to make educated, informed decisions regarding vaccinations and every other aspect of parenting. My experiences as a parent and a doctor indicate that the decision to vaccinate is no longer black or white. There are many shades in between that will set a tone that is right for your family. The information in this book is designed for parents who have chosen to vaccinate their children as well as for parents who have chosen not to. This concise guide will help you in making an informed choice regarding your child and vaccinations, and will offer alternatives for those parents seeking options other than the standard full vaccination schedule.

CHAPTER 1

The Natural Parenting

Approach to Health

In medical school we were taught about health as a state of balance, known as *homeostasis*. After being exposed to a mild illness, accident, or stress, a healthy person responds in a way that restores the body to equilibrium and maintains it. My professors taught that health was an absence of disease, which was emphasized in my classes in anatomy and physiology. For me, the study of the structure and function of the human body was important, yet failed to fully encompass a broader meaning of health. Conventional medicine regards health as an absence of symptoms: when nothing is wrong with us, we are well. In pediatrics, the state of health was measured in well child visits, which include standard guidelines of height, weight, developmental skills, and updating of shots. But what the numbers cannot tell us is how children feel and act when they are healthy.

Since I became a holistic practitioner, my scope of responsibility has expanded. I now view health as not just a state of not being sick, but as an abundance of vitality, joy, and enthusiasm. What I strive for with my children and patients is optimal health—health that encompasses our physical and emotional selves, and provides us the energy to live life to its full potential. Holistic forms of healthcare share this commitment to optimal health. They tend to the body, mind, and emotions, but also offer a more natural way of living in relationship with our environment. Enjoying good health colors how we feel, how we live, and how we relate to the world around us. For our children it can influence the foundations that are being forged in social situations, in school, and at home. It can have dramatic effects on a child's future.

As a practitioner, I encourage parents to embrace a natural parenting approach toward health. Natural parenting is *regular* parenting; it speaks to the innate, wise, and practical traditions that have been passed on through generations while incorporating the advancements of the twenty-first century: to achieve the best of both worlds. These approaches are not mutually exclusive, and when used together, they empower parents. Knowing how to act as the first line of defense against illness for your children is the best way to keep them active, happy, and healthy.

The Conventional Perspective on Illness

In our society as a whole, from our everyday conversations to advertising in the media, we are more able to discuss our aches and pains than we are to describe what it means to be healthy. We are fluent in the language of disease; we know exactly what it feels like to be sick, and we employ a complex vocabulary to describe our symptoms. In the conventional medical world, there is much fear surrounding illness. This fear is not unfounded. Before the twentieth century, due to poor nutrition, sanitation, and hygiene, many children and adults succumbed to such illnesses as smallpox, measles, tuberculosis, typhoid, and diphtheria in epidemic proportions. However, as living conditions improved in the twentieth century, many of these illnesses decreased in frequency and severity.

Now, if you are awakened in the middle of the night by the screams of your child in distress with fever and an earache, you want to be able to offer immediate relief while treating the condition. You will most likely reach for whatever medicine will suppress the symptoms and offer comfort. But while antibiotics, antihistamines, and antacids relieve the outward signs of illness, they do not treat the underlying causes. It is no coincidence that so many of the most common standard medications begin with the prefix "anti"—they work by working *against* the body.

Standard medications, also known as allopathic medicine, are designed to alleviate symptoms by manifesting the opposite condition. A runny nose is treated by drying out the nasal passages; diarrhea may be relieved by a medication that causes constipation. These drugs do make us feel better, generally by suppressing whatever symptoms are causing discomfort. The suppression of a life-threatening condition such as an asthma attack is appropriate treatment; however, prescribing daily medication for mild annoying symptoms such as chronic allergies is not always the best strategy for ensuring children's health from the holistic perspective. The medication may have unexpected side effects and it does not treat the source of the symptom.

The Holistic Perspective on Illness

Although it may sound like an oxymoron, it is a fact that healthy children get sick, as often as several times a year. Due to an immature immune system and the sharing of germs once children enter the preschool years, most of these illnesses are self-limiting, meaning they will heal on their own if untreated. Moreover, they aid in strengthening the immune system; symptoms such as runny nose, fever, and swollen glands are signs of a strong immune response. In the long run, your child's cold can mean better resistance to more severe illnesses and chronic diseases.

It is not uncommon for children to get sick at times of growth, including developmental phases such as teething and beginning to walk and speak. Illness is a natural process for the body and is part of what are called the Six Processes of Life, basic rules governing all living organisms. The six processes are growth, digestion, elimination, disease, healing, and regeneration, and they help keep us in balance, physically, mentally, and emotionally. Since disease is one of the six processes you can see why it is impossible to completely eradicate disease.

Holistic philosophy sees the human being as a complex individual comprised of mental, emotional, physical, and spiritual planes. In a healthy individual, all aspects are in balance. In contrast to standard medicine, which generally is solely preoccupied with the physical body, holistic medicine views health and illness as products of the spirit as much as the body. If our minds are distressed, our emotions in turmoil, and our environment toxic or stressful, our bodies will let us know. Holistic treatments such as Chinese medicine (including acupuncture), homeopathy, osteopathy, and other forms of natural medicine seek to restore balance by strengthening the whole person. Homeopath Dr. George Vithoulkas defines sickness as a state of imbalance, in which "stimuli are stronger than the organism's natural resistance." According to Vithoulkas, the three main causes that can lead to illness are family history, iatrogenic treatments (medications or doctor induced), and a strong stimulus such as a major accident or powerful flu virus.

Acute and Chronic Disease

Even though children get sick more often than adults, not all illnesses are created equal. There is a clear distinction. Certain sicknesses, such as self-limiting illnesses like colds, coughs, and earaches, are considered acute illnesses. Most illnesses our children experience are mild acute conditions that will respond to rest and proper nutrition. These are healthy, natural challenges for their immune systems.

In a chronic illness, the body is not able to cure itself. This can be more serious and require daily medication. In recent years, I have witnessed a dramatic increase in these sorts of conditions—monthly ear infections, severe asthma, allergies, or eczema, or even behavioral problems like Attention Deficit Hyperactivity Disorder. The explanations for the increase in chronic childhood illnesses are complex and often contradictory; the effects on children and families, however, are profound and evident.

Despite the various approaches and sometimes difference of opinion, parents can incorporate both conventional and holistic approaches in their children's lives. They are not mutually exclusive. Some families employ two practitioners—a conventional pediatrician or family doctor for well child visits and regular check-ups, and a holistic practitioner for the use of natural medicines to prevent and treat acute and chronic illnesses and to help strengthen a child's constitution. Similarly, with vaccinations, it is possible to incorporate both conventional and holistic approaches, which we will discuss in Chapter 6.

CHAPTER 2

The Immune System

and Vaccinations

In the world in which we live we are surrounded by flora and fauna that inhabit and affect our environment. On a smaller scale, microorganisms are everywhere, in our environment as well as in our bodies. Many of these organisms coexist beneficially within us, serving as the flora and fauna of our bodily habitats. Not all bacteria are healthful, however, and an imbalance of even the most beneficial microorganisms can cause infection. There are two differing theories that explain how we catch contagious illnesses like chickenpox, colds, and the flu.

The controversial nineteenth-century scientist Louis Pasteur's germ theory remains popular in the mainstream medicine community. Based on a warfare model, his theory claims that germs attack us from outside the body, causing illness; you are exposed to a bug, you get sick. On the other hand, holistic medicine recognizes that we become sick when we are in a vulnerable state; you are exposed to a bug, you get sick if you are susceptible. This latter point of view rings more true for me, for as a physician I'm in close proximity with sick people, especially in the colder months, yet it doesn't mean I am sick all the time. Several winters ago, there was a particularly severe flu epidemic in the community and I was surprised I was resistant and stayed healthy. That spring I was underdressed in the nighttime air, caught a chill, and became sick.

In general, if your child is in a weakened state, there is a higher chance of contracting whatever illness he or she is exposed to. This thinking helps to explain why only some children become ill if exposed to a sick person. How to treat these illnesses is also subject to difference of opinion. The mainstream approach, which combats illness with standard medicines, provides relief, but can also cause adverse effects, sometimes worse than the illness itself. Holistic medicine focuses on factors that can naturally strengthen the body's constitution, such as nutrition, exercise, balanced relationships, and natural medicine.

Natural Immunity

How your child gets sick after being exposed to another child who has a runny nose, fever, and cough follows a natural progression. Typically, the bacteria or virus enters through the mouth or nose (some researchers include the ear as well). The immune system becomes activated at the level of the tonsils, at which point if your child is vulnerable he or she may begin to show signs of becoming sick, such as fatigue, crankiness, or sore throat.

Once your child becomes "infected," the inflammatory process quickly begins. He or she can come down with fever, runny nose, swollen glands, and even rash, which can last from a few days to over a week. This is followed by a healing phase. This cycle—exposure, infection, inflammation, and healing—will occur over and over throughout childhood and adulthood, and does not mean that you or your child is unhealthy. Generally, these bouts of mild illnesses strengthen the immune system, making it better able to respond to bacteria or viruses in the future. If your child is sick often, talk to your practitioner about possible reasons and a treatment plan to help strengthen your child's immune system and constitution.

Passive Immunity

Throughout the day, we are continually being exposed to potentially harmful organisms and infectious germs like bacteria, viruses, parasites, and fungi. Over thousands of years, the immune system has evolved to respond by defending the body against foreign invasion. Babies are born with an immature immune system that strengthens and adapts with age. However, your child is protected through mother's antibodies that are passed through the placenta during pregnancy and in breastmilk after birth. Known as *passive immunity*, this temporary immunity can last from 6 to 12 months and beyond. For this reason, I encourage mothers to breastfeed at least a year, if not longer.

Innate and Adaptive Immune Systems

Any organism like a bacteria or virus that triggers an immune response is called an antigen. If an antigen is identified and recognized, the cells of the immune system respond by producing antibodies. Like a lock and its key, antibodies attach themselves to specific antigens. When germs are encountered, this complex chain of events unfolds in the immune system to help protect the body. Known as *natural immunity*, it is a "smart" system that has the ability to react immediately as well as to recognize and respond to germs it encountered in the past. Some illnesses your child will get once in a lifetime (chickenpox); others, such as the flu, which contain variable strains, come yearly.

The *innate immune system* is the body's first line of defense, found in the skin and mucous membranes in the mouth, nose, and gut. Innate immunity offers fast-acting cellular defense against foreign microorganisms and germs, and is the reason for symptoms such as fever, swollen glands, and runny nose. These annoying complaints are a sign that your child's immune system is effectively responding to these germs in a way that is meant to annihilate the bug and protect your child from further complications. For this reason, more practitioners are encouraging parents to view these symptoms as a normal bodily reaction that doesn't need to always be immediately counteracted with Tylenol or Motrin. In fact, many standard medications may interfere with the body's ability to effectively protect the body.

The immune system cells that circulate through the body and monitor it for harmful invaders are a group of white blood cells called leukocytes. Some of these (called lymphocytes) respond to, attack, and destroy invading organisms, while others (called phagocytes) ingest and destroy them. There are additional cells that, when activated, trigger antibodies in the body's fluids (or humors) which serve to block organisms like viruses or bacteria from spreading. If your child is not able to protect him- or herself from an invading microbe, the adaptive humoral immune system becomes activated.

The *adaptive (acquired) immune system*, also known as humoral immunity, develops over a lifetime and is more sophisticated than the innate immune system because it is able to remember, recognize, and mount an attack of antibodies against specific organisms. Once the initial lines of cellular defense are activated from the innate immune system, antibodies and other specialized immune cells such as T-cells are produced to expedite healing and also offer protection in case of future exposure. It is for this reason that children who get the chickenpox don't get it again. The adaptive immune system responds to different diseases naturally or following vaccinations.

Artificial Immunity

A vaccination is a preparation that contains a killed or weakened bacteria or virus. After injection, the adaptive humoral immune system begins a protective response. Antibodies are developed to remember, neutralize, and destroy the germs if encountered in the future. The small amount of germs is meant to stimulate the immune system without causing the actual disease. The goal with the childhood vaccination program is to protect children from many diseases without their having the illness first. For this reason it is known as *artificial immunity*.

CHAPTER 3

Pro-Vaccination and

Anti-Vaccination Viewpoints

Belief in vaccination is deep-seated in our culture, and indoctrination begins at an early age when parents with good intentions go to the pediatrician every two months in the first year for their well child check-ups and routine shots. In light of the current debates, though, many parents are questioning and researching the advantages as well as the drawbacks of the vaccine program. As Goethe wrote, "We should hear both sides quietly," and whether you choose to vaccinate or not, I believe it's important to make an informed decision based on reviewing the pro- and anti-vaccination viewpoints.

If you peruse the literature regarding vaccinations, you'll find that the statistics and points of view can vary widely depending upon your sources. A common set of statistics includes the morbidity (the incidence, or number of new cases) and mortality (the number of deaths) for each disease. It is important to know where the information used to calculate these statistics comes from, in order to evaluate how accurate each number is. When talking about vaccine effectiveness, for instance, supporters usually cite the fact that the incidence of illness is lower since the vaccine was introduced.

They typically rely upon the number of disease cases reported to the local health department to calculate the incidence of illness. However, different local health departments may have different reporting standards, and many practitioners may simply neglect to report some cases to the health department, so these figures may not be reliable. Mortality rates from a disease are generally more accurate due to higher standards in record keeping.

In general, information from mainstream agencies such as the Centers for Disease Control and Prevention (CDC) and American Academy of Pediatrics (AAP), as well as the majority of healthcare providers, is overwhelmingly in favor of the vaccine program. On the other end of the spectrum lie organizations such as the National Vaccine Information Center (NVIC), which started a vaccine safety and awareness program in the 1980s.

In a quest to do right, many parents have attempted to discuss the vaccine controversy with their doctors. Unfortunately, many doctors are unwilling to have an open discussion about shots and the current vaccine controversy, often because they are similarly confused. To help dispel vaccination myths and to guide you in finding the most accurate information about vaccines, the following is a summary of the main topics of contention between advocates ("Pro-Vaccination Viewpoint") and critics ("Anti-Vaccination Viewpoint") of vaccinations.

The benefits of vaccines outweigh the risk.

PRO-VACCINATION VIEWPOINT: The benefits of vaccines greatly outweigh the risks, and the shots are relatively innocuous compared to the severity of the illnesses. Like any medication, vaccines can carry the risk of adverse effects, but they are rare. Most children experience no side effects or occasionally mild complaints of fussiness, slight fever, or soreness at the site of the shot. Not to vaccinate places a child at risk of contracting a potentially serious or deadly illness that could have been prevented.

ANTI-VACCINATION VIEWPOINT: We are being inundated with numerous personal accounts that link the shots to serious illnesses, even death. Many parents believe that vaccinations pose serious risks to children and are by no means completely safe, and on this side of the argument it is widely believed that the risks do not outweigh the benefits.

COMMENTS: Both opinions appear to present valid points of view. On the pro-vaccination side, children should not have to suffer these illnesses, especially if they are preventable by immunization, and most children tolerate the shots without a problem. I feel that this opinion is not entirely true, because we know that it is impossible to eliminate disease altogether. Although fewer children are having chickenpox, mumps, or rubella, I believe that the increase in chronic diseases can be linked at least in part to vaccinations and overuse of medications, including antibiotics. Also, although the risk of adverse effects may be rare for most children, it is very real. Although I recognize the severity of some of the illnesses, it is important to weigh the benefits and risks of each illness and corresponding vaccination in order to make a decision about each vaccination. If you choose not to vaccinate, then it is especially important for you to know how to prevent and treat that illness. If you choose to vaccinate, then use the Safe Shot Strategy in Chapter 7 to prevent or minimize side effects.

Vaccines are responsible for the decline of serious childhood diseases.

PRO-VACCINATION VIEWPOINT: The decline and eradication of many serious childhood illnesses are a result of the vaccination program. Illnesses that were frequent in the past are nowhere near as common now and supporters consider mass immunization a monumental achievement in public health in the twentieth century. Before vaccinations, many severe illnesses occurred in epidemic proportions and countless children and adults died during outbreaks of such diseases as diphtheria, smallpox, and the measles.

For example, in the 1940s there were thousands of cases of diphtheria in the United States, while currently there are less than five reported cases a year. Once a minimum of 75 percent of children are vaccinated in a community, the probability of the disease occurring in epidemic proportions decreases. This phenomenon is called *herd immunity*, and can prevent the spread of disease even to children who are not immunized. Unvaccinated children lower the herd immunity and increase the risk of those illnesses returning in epidemic proportions.

ANTI-VACCINATION VIEWPOINT: Critics acknowledge that the vaccination program has influenced the rate of decline of childhood illnesses; however, many of these illnesses had already begun to decrease in incidence as well as severity before mandatory vaccines were introduced. Many attribute this to general improvements in nutrition, sanitation, refrigeration of food, and standards in medical care as well as natural changes in disease cycles. According to the British Association for the Advancement of Science, diseases of childhood had decreased up to 90 percent between 1850 and 1940. For example, the rate of diphtheria began to decrease before the vaccine was developed in the 1920s, and the mortality rate went from 86 percent to less than 10 percent in the past one hundred years.

In some instances, statistics were altered in order to give the impression to the public of the effectiveness of the vaccines. With regards to polio, by the time the vaccine was introduced in the mid-1950s, the epidemic had already begun to wane. In a 1962 U.S congressional hearing, the head of the Department of Biostatistics of the University of North Carolina School of Public Health testified that the number of polio cases had increased following the vaccination. To present the polio vaccine in a favorable light, the statistic were altered. To further support the campaign, the number of cases that constitute an epidemic as well as the classification of the polio disease were reformulated following the launching of the polio vaccine program. This means that after the vaccine was introduced a grerater number of polio cases were needed to be considered an epidemic. Also, diseases similar to polio, such as Guillain-Barré Syndrome, were no longer considered to be polio cases but were counted as a separate illness.

COMMENTS: Both points of view are convincing. Although many of the illnesses have decreased due to the vaccines, many were on the decline before the vaccine programs were begun. From the holistic point of view, I believe that certain illnesses in childhood are a fact of life. Most healthy children heal from the illness without complications and are provided with lifetime immunity. When my sons came down with chickenpox, I was relieved they got it in childhood and not as adults when it could be more severe.

The mass vaccination program has led to a rise in chronic disease among children.

PRO-VACCINATION VIEWPOINT: The media hype about the possible links of vaccinations to chronic diseases such asthma, autism, or ADHD are unfounded, and cause unnecessary fear among parents. According to the CDC, getting the vaccine is much safer than getting the disease. If a vaccinated child does get the disease, it is usually a mild form. In the case of chickenpox, before the mass vaccination program, 12,000 people were hospitalized for complications and there were 100 deaths each year. If a vaccinated child does get the chickenpox, it is often a milder form of the disease.

ANTI-VACCINATION VIEWPOINT: Over the past several decades, there has been a shift in childhood illnesses. Compared with when I was growing up in the 1960s and 70s, children are being immunized for a wider array of diseases and the number of immunizations has increased from 8 to 30. Acute illnesses like chickenpox are much less common, but more children are being treated for chronic diseases and disabilities, which are increasing in epidemic proportions. Since the mid-twentieth century, mental illnesses and neurological diseases have quadrupled, learning disorders are up 1,000 times, and allergies, asthma, and ear infections are now chronic childhood conditions. While studies have yet to definitively link vaccines to these more unusual illnesses, researchers are beginning to question the role of vaccines in neurocognitive disorders like autism, Asperger's, and ADHD, and diseases like asthma and leukemia.

Researchers from a study of over 1,200 children at the Wellington School of Medicine, New Zealand, compared the rates of asthma in vaccinated versus unvaccinated children. The immunized children had 22.5 percent asthma consultations and 30 percent consultations for other allergic illness. Unvaccinated children (no DTP or polio shots) had no history of medical consultations for asthma or allergic conditions. There have been instances where children who had chronic conditions such as asthma or eczema were cured after episodes of whooping cough or measles respectively. This suggests a positive role the childhood illnesses may play in prevention of chronic illnesses.

COMMENTS: Having seen the increase in chronic conditions and neurological disorders in my own practice, I am convinced that many of these illnesses in children may be linked to increased vaccination. However, I believe that lifestyle, environment, nutrition, antibiotics, and other factors also play a role. In a patient population that is approximately 50 percent vaccinated, I have treated a small number of unvaccinated children with many of the same illnesses.

A vaccine is prepared in such a way that it is similar to the illness but not dangerous.

PRO-VACCINATION VIEWPOINT: Vaccines are made according to maximum safety standards. In order to manufacture a vaccination, the bacteria and viruses must be prepared in a way that stimulates a proper immune response most effectively without causing harm. The most common types of vaccines currently being used are inactivated (killed) or live. Inactivated vaccines consist of killed microorganisms and take longer to stimulate an immune response. To make them more effective, substances called adjuvants are added to the preparation to enhance the immune response. Aluminum compounds are commonly used as adjuvants. Flu, hepatitis A and B, pertussis, and polio shots are examples of inactivated vaccines. Diphtheria and tetanus vaccines are inactivated toxoids, made from the harmful toxic substance, not from the organism itself. Because the microorganisms are inactivated and take longer to trigger an immune response, booster shots are often recommended.

Live vaccines contain an attenuated (weakened) live strain of the microorganism, and offer a longer-lasting immune defense compared to the inactivated vaccines. Although the germ is considered sufficiently modified, it is possible to get a mild case of the disease. The measles, mumps, and rubella (MMR) shot consists of live virus strains. In general, live vaccines are usually not recommended for pregnant women.

In addition to the inactivated and live forms of vaccinations, there are other preparations being used. The hepatitis B vaccine is a subunit vaccine that contains fragments of a germ. It is made in yeast and consists of the surface proteins of the virus. *Haemophilus influenzae* type B vaccine is a conjugate vaccine in which the outer layer of the bacteria is combined with a protein to stimulate an immune response.

ANTI-VACCINATION VIEWPOINT: There are many instances where children have suffered serious reactions to a vaccination. In inactive vaccines, even killed microorganizations and toxoids can be harmful. Pertussis bacteria used in the whooping cough vaccine produce toxins that can be harmful to the brain and cause convulsions similar to the illness, making it hard to tell whether a negative reaction following a shot is the result of faulty preparation. The adjuvants, such as aluminum, used in the preparation of many inactivated vaccines can also cause reactions in the body such as pain, redness, or swelling around the site of the shot as well as vague symptoms of nausea, drowsiness, and weakness.

In live vaccinations, even weak germs can sometimes cause disease. The live oral polio vaccine was discontinued when it was discovered that it caused more cases of paralytic polio than the actual disease. Although the germs in the live virus MMR vaccine are considered sufficiently modified, it is possible to get a mild case of the disease from the vaccine.

COMMENTS: Although the bacteria and viruses used have been slightly altered, a vaccine can have possible harmful effects that come from either the organism itself or the preservatives and chemicals. Also, since vaccines are administered as a shot, you are injecting these organisms and chemicals directly into the bloodstream, bypassing the body's normal defenses. For this reason, if you are going to vaccinate, make sure your child is in good health with a strong immune system.

Vaccination is different from having the disease and competes with the body's natural immune system.

PRO-VACCINATION VIEWPOINT: The vaccine is meant to create a similar reaction to having a natural illness. Once the bacteria or virus is injected into the body, an immune response is activated that protects the child. In some instances it is only for a period of time; for that reason, boosters are given periodically.

ANTI-VACCINATION VIEWPOINT: Naturally acquired illnesses usually occur one at a time. By giving shots that may contain four to six bacteria and viruses at once, we could be overstimulating the immune system. Could you imagine your child having diphtheria, whooping cough, and meningitis at the same time? Vaccinations often recreate a similar situation in your child's body.

A vaccine is meant to trick the body into thinking it is being exposed, yet the natural routes (through the mouth, nose, and intestine) are bypassed and the bacteria or virus is injected directly into the bloodstream. The injections thus circumvent the body's natural defense mechanism and may contribute to the rise of chronic diseases in children. Because vaccines grant an artificial immunity that is often temporary and not sustainable, many people do not consider them immunizations at all. Each year new research emerges, and we still do not fully understand the ramifications of vaccinations on the immune system and beyond.

COMMENTS: Among holistic medical practitioners, many believe that common childhood illnesses help the immune system to mature and become stronger, making it more effective in dealing with challenges from viruses and bacteria later in life. This kind of natural immunity lasts longer and in many cases is lifelong. Vaccinations do not offer lifetime immunity, and instead shift the illness to vulnerable adults who are susceptible to a more dangerous version of the disease. Chickenpox during adulthood, for instance, is a risky disease, presenting far more complications than the childhood version. When my sons had chickenpox, I was humbled by the suffering my 11-year-old son experienced. Although I wished I could alleviate my son's discomfort from the rash, I also had to acknowledge that vaccines can have side effects just as uncomfortable as—and sometimes more harmful than—the illnesses they prevent. I have witnessed the tragedies that have occurred following a shot, and provided care to many children who have responded poorly to vaccination.

It is more important to vaccinate the entire population regardless of need.

PRO-VACCINATION VIEWPOINT: The goal of public health officials is to consider the health needs of children and offer protection through mass vaccination. It is easier to provide the same routine vaccinations for all children.

ANTI-VACCINATION VIEWPOINT: Many opponents have criticized the one-size-fits-all compulsory approach to vaccination that doesn't consider an individual child's needs. For instance, the hepatitis B shot is recommended for infants following birth. Hepatitis B is considered a sexually transmitted illness and not a childhood disease. The only children at risk for contracting hepatitis B are those born to high-risk mothers who have a history of hepatitis B, which can stem from a blood transfusion, intravenous drug abuse, or prostitution. When one mother who had no history of hepatitis B and was not in a high-risk category questioned her pediatrician about the value of this shot, he replied that it was possible that the child could come into contact with a dirty needle at the park. Based on his reply, the mother refused the shot and stated that she would consider the vaccine in the future when her child was approaching the teen years.

COMMENTS: When possible, it is always best to consider an individual's needs, strengths, and susceptibilities in all aspects of healthcare. The rationale for some of the mandated shots seem superfluous and questionable (for example, hepatitis A usually has no symptoms in children).

Mercury toxicity is no longer an issue.

PRO-VACCINATION VIEWPOINT: Mercury has been used as a preservative since the 1930s, and is known commercially as thimerosal (trade name: Rithialate). This is an antibacterial compound that contains 50 percent ethyl mercury. Because it has received a lot of attention regarding possible health risks, mercury has apparently been removed from most vaccines.

ANTI-VACCINATION VIEWPOINT: Many vaccines are currently mercury-free; however, there are still lots that contain trace levels of mercury. The following shots contained mercury in the past and currently may still contain trace amounts: DTaP, Hib, and hepatitis B. The MMR, polio, and chickenpox vaccines never had mercury.

In addition, there is a phenomenon that occurs when mercury is combined with aluminum, another common vaccine additive. Scientists found that when mercury and aluminum were used together in laboratory animals, the dangerous effects and mortality rates were greatly increased, causing a *synergistic toxicity*. Mercury can be dangerous to the brain and kidney; high levels are known to cause tics, speech delay, sleep disorders, attention deficit disorder, and autism. It is ironic that the FDA advises that pregnant women avoid mercury-laden fish like shark, mackerel, swordfish, and tilefish, while the flu vaccine, which is known to contain mercury, is recommended to be given to pregnant women.

In 1991, a memo from the executives at the pharmaceutical company Merck acknowledged that by the time a child is six months old, he or she could receive an accumulated dose of mercury that is up to 87 times higher than guidelines given for the maximum daily consumption of mercury from fish. The younger the infant or fetus is when exposed to mercury, the greater the possibility for health risks, and studies have shown the mercury levels increase according to the number of shots a child has received containing mercury.

Most childhood vaccination schedules exceed the federal guidelines on acceptable levels of ingested mercury. As a precaution, vaccine manufacturers have been asked to voluntarily limit their use of thimerosal. The organization Health Advocacy in the Public Interest (HAPI) tested four vaccines for heavy metals. According to HAPI, "The June 2004 lab results from Doctor's Data run counter to vaccine manufacturers' claims. For example, some product inserts currently claim that a 'trace' amount of mercury still exists in the final product but that the amount has been greatly reduced. Others claim to be producing completely mercury-free products. All four vaccine vials tested contained mercury despite manufacturer claims that two of the vials were completely mercury-free. All four vials also contained aluminum; one contained nine times more than the other three, tremendously enhancing the toxicity of mercury which causes neuronal death in the brain."

COMMENTS: When we purchase vaccinations for our office, whenever possible we attempt to get thimerosal-free vaccines in single-dose vials or individual pre-filled syringes. In general, most physicians use the larger multi-dose vials because they are more cost-effective and easier to store. However, these multi-dose vials contain preservatives to prevent contamination after the vial is opened.

Even though mercury toxicity may no longer be as much of an issue, many vaccines still contain trace amounts of mercury. Plus, I do not believe it is the only harmful component used; there are other culprits listed such as aluminum, formaldehyde, and lye.

The additives, preservatives, and other inactive ingredients (mercury, in particular) are safe in the small amounts used in vaccines.

PRO-VACCINATION VIEWPOINT: The manufacturing process of a vaccine involves necessary excipients (inactive ingredients) which help stabilize, preserve, and enhance the solution. Vaccine advocates believe they are given in such minute amounts that they are not a cause for concern in humans.

ANTI-VACCINATION VIEWPOINT: There are no safe levels of many of these additives, which are known to be toxic chemicals, or poisons, or to have cancer-causing (carcinogenic) properties. In laboratory testing of animals, many excipients are known to be dangerous in high enough doses, as the table below indicates.

COMMENTS: It is unfortunate that many toxic additives are needed in the preparation of the vaccines. Even if they are used in small amounts, some children can be affected by the additives, which may affect children who have allergies to antibiotics, egg, or gelatin.

Some of the vaccine components such as aborted human tissue raise ethical issues.

PRO-VACCINATION VIEWPOINT: Like medications, vaccinations have gone through rigorous trials and approval strategies that sometimes require testing on laboratory animals and use of tissue from human and other animal sources. They are intended for the good of mankind and improve the lives of millions of children and adults.

ANTI-VACCINATION VIEWPOINT: The use of aborted human fetuses, pigs, and other animal sources raises ethical, religious, and moral questions among many families. Some vaccines are manufactured from the cells of aborted human fetuses. For instance, MRC-5 cellular protein comes from the lung tissue of a 14-week-old male fetus and is used in the hepatitis A, hepatitis B, polio, and varicella vaccines. In the 1960s, the WI-38 (Wistar Institute 38) was produced from an aborted female fetus and was used in the rubella and varicella shots. In addition, gelatin and vaccine culture media are sometimes made from cows, pigs, chickens, and monkeys, which may pose significant health hazards. The culture media listed in the chart are used in the preparation of the vaccines.

COMMENTS: Crossing species lines by using animal components could cause pathogenic strains that can be formed with unknown long-term adverse effects. Monkey tissue used in preparation of the polio vaccine, for instance, has been known to be contaminated with the simian virus 40 (SV40). Initially thought to be harmless, SV40 has been linked to cancer.

VACCINE CULTURE MEDIA	VACCINE
Bovine	DTaP, DTaP-HepB-IPV Polio, Pneumococcal
Chick embryo	Influenza, Measles, Mumps,
Chick kidney cells	Influenza
Human diploid tissue culture MRC-5	Hepatitis A, Hepatitis B, Polio Varicella
Human diploid tissue culture WI-38	Rubella, Varicella
Monkey kidney tissue	Polio

INACTIVE INGREDIENTS IN VACCINES

INACTIVE INGREDIENT	USES	VACCINE	ADVERSE EFFECTS
Albumin, human serum	Stabilizer, growth medium	Measles Mumps, Rubella, MMR	Fever, nausea, vomiting, and allergic reactions including rash, hives, itching.
Albumin or serum, bovine, Fetal Bovine Serum (FBS)	Stabilizer, growth medium	Hepatitis A, MMR Measles, Mumps, Rubella, Varicella (chickenpox)	May be contaminated with nanobacteria and a pestivirus called bovine viral diarrhea virus. No known positive effects. Complications are being researched.
Aluminum hydroxide	Adjuvant	Anthrax, DTaP, DT, Td, Hib, Hepatitis B, Hepatitis A	A well-known connection between the use of aluminum and Alzheimer's disease. According to neuroscientist Chris Shaw, possibly linked to symptoms associated with Parkinson's, amyotrophic lateral sclerosis (ALS, or Lou Gehrig's disease), dementia, and Alzheimer's. Irritating reactions at the site of injections such as inflammation, swelling, and redness.
Aluminum phosphate	Adjuvant	DTaP, Td, Pneumococcal (Prevnar), Hepatitis A, Hepatitis B	Skin irritation and burns. Nausea, vomiting, diarrhea, and shock. Damage to kidneys and liver.
Aluminum potassium sulfate	Adjuvant	DTaP, DT	Irritation of skin, eyes, and respiratory tract. Nausea, vomiting and diarrhea.

INACTIVE INGREDIENT	USES	VACCINE	ADVERSE EFFECTS
Amino acids	Growth medium	Anthrax, Hepatitis A, Hepatitis B, Td	Building blocks of protein, and play an important role in various functions of the body. Toxicity caused by the injection of amino acids into the bloodstream from vaccinations may be linked to abnormal immune responses in children with developmental delays and autism.
Ammonium sulfate	Protein fractionation	Hib	Eye, skin, respiratory irritant. Toxic to gastrointestinal tract, liver, and brain.
Bactopeptone	Growth medium	Influenza	Associated with estrogen-like activity. Estrogen, an important hormone, can have deleterious effects on female secondary sex characteristics such as breast growth in young children.
Beta propiolactone (propiolactone)	Viral inactivator, disinfectant, sterilizer	Influenza	Severe irritant. Considered a hazardous chemical. Causes breathing difficulty, severe blistering and burns of the skin and eyes with contact. According to the *Second Annual Report on Carcinogens*, propiolactone was initially listed in 1981 as "reasonably expected to be a human carcinogen." (IARC 1999)

INACTIVE INGREDIENT	USES	VACCINE	ADVERSE EFFECTS
Benzethonium chloride	Preservative, antiseptic, antibacterial, anti-infective	Anthrax	Powerful chemical that blocks neuromuscular transmission. Considered harmful if swallowed, inhaled, or absorbed through the skin. Can lead to serious damage to the eyes.
DNA (human)	Manufacturing residue	Hepatitis A	DNA mutation can happen spontaneously or be caused by radiation, UV light, chemicals, or viruses and has been linked to some cancers. Injection of foreign DNA into the body does not have any positive known effects, and may be deleterious over the long-term.
EDTA (ethyl-enediamine-tetraacetic acid)	Preservative	Varicellla (chickenpox)	Corrosive liquid causing irritation. Toxic to kidney, liver, and lungs.
Egg protein	Manufacturing residue, growth medium	Influenza, Yellow Fever	Allergic reactions to egg protein include nausea, headache, stomachache, difficulty breathing, hives, and drop in blood pressure. Discuss with your practitioner if your child has a reaction to eggs, chicken, or chicken feathers.
Formalde-hyde, formalin	Preservative, anti-microbial	Anthrax, DTaP, DT, Td, Hib, Hepatitis A, Hepatitis B, Influenza, Polio	Causes burns. May be toxic to kidney, cause allergic reactions, cause cancer to humans. Possible genetic damage.

INACTIVE INGREDIENT	USES	VACCINE	ADVERSE EFFECTS
Porcine Gelatin	Stabilizer	DTaP, Influenza, MMR, Measles, Mumps, Rubella, Varicella, Yellow Fever	Many cause severe allergic reactions including hives, low blood pressure, runny nose, and faintness.
Gentamicin	Anti-bacterial	Influenza (FluMist)	Antibiotic with known toxicity to the ear vestibular apparatus, causing disturbances in balance and hearing and kidney damage. Also linked to diarrhea, twitching, and seizures.
Glutaraldehyde	Toxin detoxifier	DtaP, DtaP, Hepatitis B, Polio	Exposure causes headaches, drowsiness, dizziness, and irritation to eyes, skin, and respiratory system.
Hydrochloric acid	Adjusts pH	DTaP, DT	Extremely corrosive. May be fatal if ingested. Damages skin and eyes.
Lactose	Stabilizer	Hib, Meningoccocal	More commonly seen as a food allergy, symptoms include vomiting, diarrhea, constipation, rash, hives, and wheezing.
Mercury (see page 25)			
Monosodium glutamate (MSG)	Stabilizer, preservative	Influenza (FluMist), Varicella	May cause headache, dizziness, and chest pain.
MRC-5 cellular protein (Lung tissue of male fetus)	Manufacturing residue, growth medium	Hepatitis A, Hepaitis B, Polio, Varicella	From the lung tissue of an aborted male fetus, which contains DNA, protein, and cells. The use of tissue as well as the risk of contamination have no known positive effects and may be deleterious in the longterm.

INACTIVE INGREDIENT	USES	VACCINE	ADVERSE EFFECTS
Neomycin	Antibiotic	DTap, Hepatitis A, Hepatitis B, Influenza, MMR, Measles, Mumps, Rubella, Polio, Varicella	Side effects when taken orally are rash, diarrhea, nausea, vomiting, colitis, and damage to the kidney and ears.
Phenol	Preservative, antibacterial	Pneumococcal	Systemic poison. Burns. Toxic if inhaled.
2-Phen-oxyethanol	Preservative	DTaP, Hepatitis A, Hepatitis B, Polio Td	Harmful if swallowed or absorbed through the skin.
Phosphate buffers	Adjust pH	DTaP, DT, Hib, Hepatitis A, Hepatitis B, Influenza (Flu-Mist), MMR, Measles, Mumps, Rubella, Polio Varicella	Harmful if inhaled, ingested, or absorbed into the skin. Can cause irritation to eyes, ears, respiratory tract, and skin, and may affect kidneys, heart, and brain.
Polyethylene glycol p-isooctyl-phenyl ether (Triton X-100)	Viral inactivation	Influenza	Harmful if swallowed or inhaled, or contacts skin. May contain traces of ethylene oxide, probably cancer-causing to humans.
Polymyxin B	Antibacterial	DTaP, Hepatitis B, Influenza, Polio	May be toxic to brain and kidneys.
Polyoxy-ethylene 9-10 nonylphenol (Octoxynol 9)	Viral inactivator	Influenza	Known as a vaginal spermicide; the side effects include local allergic reactions and irritation.
Polysorbate 20 (Tween® 20)	Surfactant	Hepatitis A, Hepatitis B	Can cause irritation to skin and eyes.

INACTIVE INGREDIENT	USES	VACCINE	ADVERSE EFFECTS
Polysorbate 80 (Tween® 80)	Surfactant	DTaP, Hepatitis B, HPV, Polio	Can cause eye irritation and anaphylactic reactions. Has been linked to infertility in mice.
Sodium acetate	Stabilizer	DT, Td	Harmful if ingested, swallowed, or absorbed through skin.
Sodium bisulfite	Preservative	Influenza	Harmful if swallowed or ingested. May cause allergic reactions, especially in asthmatics.
Sodium borate	Adjusts pH	Hepatitis A, Hepatitis B, Hib	Harmful if swallowed, inhaled, or absorbed in the skin. In high doses, may cause coughing, shortness of breath, muscle spasm, kidney damage, shock, coma, and death.
Sodium chloride	Adjusts tonicity	DTaP, DT, Td, MMR, Measles, Mumps, Rubella, Polio, Varicella	May cause skin, eye, or respiratory irritation.
Sodium hydroxide (lye)	Adjusts pH	DT, Td	Toxic if ingested. Corrosive. Severe burns.
Sorbitol	Stabilizer, solvent	Measles, Mumps, Rubella, MMR	Commonly used as a sugar substitute in diet foods. May be associated with rash, itching, swelling, nausea, gas, diarrhea, cramps, and anal irritation. Parents are advised to use caution with children who may be more sensitive to its effects.

INACTIVE INGREDIENT	USES	VACCINE	ADVERSE EFFECTS
Streptomycin	Antibiotic	Influenza, Polio	Nausea, vomiting, dizziness, rash and fever.
Sucrose	Stabilizer	Hib, Influenza (FluMist), Hib, Measles, Mumps, MMR, Varicella	Common table sugar. Linked to obesity, insulin resistance, hypoglycemia, and diabetes. Many children are sensitive to sugar in their diet.
Tributylphosphate	Viral inactivator	Influenza	Causes burns with possible brain effects. May be carcinogenic or mutagenic, or have reproductive effects.

CHAPTER 4

The Role of Government, Pharmaceutical Companies, and Insurance

The days of the early apothecary shops displaying mortars, pestles, herbs, and roots have given way to the pharmaceutical industry. The strength of the drug companies was fueled by the discovery and mass production of insulin by the 1920s and penicillin by the 1940s. Over the decades, more medications have been mass produced and made available to the public. The pharmaceutical companies have expanded in wealth and power with the ability to exert tremendous clout throughout the world to their advantage. With the large amount of influence, laws have been passed that attempt to enforce guidelines regarding the testing, approval, and labeling of drugs, including vaccinations.

The drug companies have been accused of conflict of interest and deceptive promotions. Amidst the successes of such medications as "The Pill" came the tragedies. From 1957 to 1961, thalidomide, a tranquilizer, was commonly prescribed to pregnant women to help combat morning sickness; sadly, however, thalidomide caused severe birth defects in these women's children. More recently, Merck released the pain medication Vioxx, even though, according to the Alliance for Human Research Protection, some internal studies showed that some users might have an increased risk of heart disease.

Vaccine manufacturers have also been accused of conflict of interest. Members of advisory committees on vaccination and immunization policies to both the Food and Drug Administration (FDA) and the Centers for Disease Control and Prevention (CDC) have had significant ties to the drug companies, and are not supposed to participate in making decisions in which there is a financial interest to be gained. Yet there has been evidence that some members of the CDC advisory committee who sit on the vaccine approval panels also have financial ties to various pharmaceutical companies.

As a result, the FDA and CDC, which are supposed to regulate pharmaceutical companies, have been accused of being lax, with weak enforcement. According to the federal laws governing these committees, members should disclose financial agreements and those with a conflict of interest should not participate in the decision making process; the committees should have a balanced representation in terms of points of view. In 1999, the Committee on Government Reform investigated federal vaccine policies and found the CDC routinely provided waivers from conflict of interest to its members. At the center of one of the controversies was the rotavirus vaccine, which was withdrawn from the market after reports linking it to intussusception, a serious bowel obstruction requiring surgery. Following an investigation by the Committee on Government Reforms (U.S. House of Representatives, June 2000), it was found that the members on the vaccine panel who approved RotaShield had conflicts of interest. Since then, a new vaccine, RotaTeq, has been approved for prevention of rotavirus.

On April 6, 2000, the U.S. House of Representatives Government Reform Committee, chaired by Congressman Dan Burton, a Republican from Indiana, held a day of hearings to look at the possibility that vaccines could cause autism. Burton has been outspoken against vaccinations as he believes his grandson's diagnosis of autism was linked to the shots. During the hearing, ethical questions were raised about a member of the Advisory Committee on Immunization Practices (ACIP) who was a pediatrician, helped develop the rotavirus vaccine, and pressed to have mandatory vaccines at a previous symposium. The physician admitted to "apparent conflict of interest."

In addition to conflict of interest, pharmaceutical companies have been accused of presenting misleading information. In 2002, Merck was still distributing hepatitis B vaccines with mercury even though they had announced four years earlier that their line of pediatric vaccines were free from mercury.

Vaccine Adverse Event Reporting System (VAERS) and "Hot Lots"

In 1982, the National Vaccine Information Center (NVIC) became the first consumer organization promoting vaccine safety. Their mission statement says that they are "dedicated to the prevention of vaccine injuries and deaths through public education and to defending the informed consent ethic." The NVIC was originally founded by parents whose children were injured by or died from the DPT (diphtheria, pertussis, tetanus) shot. Barbara Loe Fisher, co-founder and president of the NVIC, was instrumental in organizing a vaccine safety movement in the early 1980s after her eldest son was diagnosed with multiple learning disabilities and attention deficit disorder following his fourth DPT shot at 2½ years old.

Congress passed the National Childhood Vaccine Injury Act of 1986 in response to the growing concern among parents linking vaccinations to illnesses including autism. This ensured that a healthcare provider who administers a vaccination will permanently record the date of administration, manufacturer, and lot number of the vaccine. The practitioner would also be required by law to report vaccine reactions to a central organization. From this, the U.S. government Vaccine Adverse Events Reporting System (VAERS) database operated by the FDA made possible for practitioners, parents, and vaccine manufacturers to report adverse effects from vaccines.

It is estimated that as few as 1 to 10 percent are being reported by health-care providers. In addition, adverse effects can also be reported to the NVIC. The NVIC started tracking lot numbers of DPT in 1990, and found over 90 families had reported severe reactions from the same lot number. According to the NVIC, the organization presented the findings on three different occasions to government advisory committees. No significant measures were taken.

A vaccine lot is considered a "hot lot" when associated with high numbers of complaints of injuries and deaths. The information is available at the Vaccine Adverse Event Reporting System (VAERS) database on the Internet.

The old rotavirus vaccine, RotaShield, was taken off the market because a significant number of adverse effects were reported. The jury is out on the newly marketed RotaTeq; extensive information on its effects is not available.

National Vaccine Injury Compensation Program (VICP)

The National Vaccine Injury Compensation Program (VICP), known as the vaccine court, was established in 1988 and protects the vaccine companies. It's subsidized by a surcharge on vaccines sold. The VICP is a government-run agency that provides a no-fault compensation plan for people who have been injured or killed by a vaccine reaction. It prevents suits against vaccine manufacturers. The compensation for damages from a vaccine injury or death pays up to $250,000 and must be filed within a specific period of time following injury or death.

Although the program was intended to make processing claims quick and easy for everyone, claims are sometimes held up for years and many legitimate claims are denied assistance. The guidelines have been amended over the years. This has made it more difficult for petitioners, some of whom need ongoing assistance and therapy. According to Representative Burton, the program "was supposed to be non-adversarial and it's become very adversarial. [Many people have] had legitimate claims and they went on for eight, nine, ten years." The core of the problem is that very few doctors acknowledge that vaccines can cause injuries or death.

Medical Insurance Coverage

Vaccinations are meant to be available to all children regardless of socio-economic background, either through government assistance or in the private sector. In the United States, more than half of the vaccinations are funded through public health agencies at the federal, state, or local level. Although most private and public insurance companies provide immunization benefits, they can vary depending on type of insurance, deductibles, and individual vaccines. For example, Gardasil, the vaccine for the human papillomavirus against cervical cancer, is expensive and may not be covered by all insurance plans.

Parallel to inflation and soaring medical and insurance costs, the price of vaccines is also on the rise. The American Academy of Pediatrics (AAP) has been concerned that the higher fees, along with lesser insurance benefits, will lead to under-immunization in the United States. Vaccinations are a source of income for pediatricians, who are among the lowest paid of medical specialties. In addition, according to most pediatricians, insurance coverage and reimbursements on pediatric patient visits and vaccinations are insufficient. According to Jon R. Almquist, M.D., FAAP, chair of the AAP Task Force on Immunization, "Pediatricians are not looking to make huge profits off vaccines. We're in pediatrics because we care about children but we shouldn't be expected to subsidize the public health system and perform our jobs at a loss. We've carried this burden for long enough."

CHAPTER 5

Childhood and Adolescent Vaccines and Recommended Immunization Schedule

Advertisements and commercials abound about the latest new drugs available. Although we are also provided with the list of unwanted side effects that may affect certain people, the consumer is led to believe that the benefits of the medications outweigh the risks.

Patients and parents can learn more about these medications, including vaccinations, from the *Physicians' Desk Reference* (PDR), a compilation of package inserts of thousands of prescription medicines. Issued by the Food and Drug Administration (FDA), the package insert is a handout provided at the time of vaccination and contains information in a standard format about the vaccine, its intended use, ingredients, dosages, side effects, and contraindications (who should not be given the vaccine). Many parents are disturbed to find detailed lists of adverse effects, including notices that the vaccines have not been evaluated for their carcinogenic (cancer causing) or mutagenic potential, or their potential to impair fertility.

The Recommended Immunization Schedule is published annually to provide practitioners with guidelines on the recommended ages for childhood and adult vaccinations. It is reviewed by a group of 15 immunization experts on the Advisory Committee on Immunization Practices (ACIP), part of the U.S. government. They advise the Secretary of Health and Human Services, the Assistant Secretary for Health, and the Centers for Disease Control and Prevention on the vaccine dosages, contraindications, periodicity to ensure a current and updated schedule.

In this chapter, I review each of the vaccines in the Recommended Immunization Schedule, describing the effects of both the diseases and the vaccines intended to prevent them. I attempt to give you some idea of how to gauge your child's risk of getting each illness and developing complications, as well as his or her risk for adverse side effects from the vaccine. I also summarize the conventional allopathic treatments for each illness. In addition to these treatments, there are homeopathic and natural remedies available to treat and prevent almost all of these conditions. Because homeopathic treatments are not "one size fits all," I have not listed those remedies here. If you are interested in learning more about homeopathic and natural remedies for these illnesses, please see my book *Natural Baby and Childcare*. These vaccines are presented in the order in which they are listed in the schedules on the following pages.

In addition to the vaccines in the Recommended Immunization Schedule, I describe some additional vaccines that are available, some of which may make sense if you are traveling abroad with your child.

FIGURE 1. Recommended immunization schedule for persons aged 0-6 years — United States, 2007

Vaccine	Birth	1 month	2 months	4 months	6 months	12 months	15 months	18 months	19-23 months	2-3 years	4-6 years
Hepatitis B[1]	HepB	HepB		See footnote 1		HepB				Hep B Series	
Rotavirus[2]			Rota	Rota	Rota						
Diptheria, Tetanus, Pertussis[3]			DTaP	DTaP	DTaP		DTaP				DTaP
Haemophilus Influenzae type b[4]			Hib	Hib	Hib[4]	Hib					
Pneumococcal[5]			PCV	PCV	PCV	PCV				PCV PPV	
Inactivated Poliovirus			IPV	IPV	IPV						IPV
Influenza[6]					Influenza (Yearly)						
Measles, Mumps, Rubella[7]						MMR					MMR
Varicella[8]						Varicella					Varicella
Hepatitis A[9]						HepA (2 doses)				HepA Series	
Meningococcal[10]										MPSV4	

Range of recommended ages

Catch-up immunization

Certain high-risk groups

This schedule indicates the recommended ages for routine administration of currently licensed childhood vaccines, as of December 1, 2006, for children aged 0-6 years. Additional information is available at http://www.cdc.gov/nip/recs/child-schedule.htm. Any dose not administered at the recommended age should be administered at any subsequent visit, when indicated and feasible. Additional vaccines may be licensed and recommended during the year. Licensed combination vaccines may be used whenever any components of the combination are indicated and other components of the vaccine are not contraindicated and if approved by the Food and Drug Administration for that dose of the series. Providers should consult the respective Advisory Committee on Immunization Practices statement for detailed recommendations. Clinically significant adverse events that follow immunization should be reported to the Vaccine Adverse Event Reporting System (VAERS). Guidance about how to obtain and complete a VAERS form is available at http://www.vaers.hhs.gov or by telephone, 800-822-7967.

1. **Hepatitis B vaccine (HepB).** *(Minimum age: birth)*
   At birth:
   - Administer monovalent HepB to all newborns before hospital discharge.
   - If mother is hepatitis surface antigen (HBsAG)-positive, administer HepB and 0.5 mL of hepatitis B immune globulin (HBIG) within 12 hours of birth.
   - If mother's HBsAg status is unknown, administer HepB within 12 hours of birth. Determine the HBsAg status as soon as possible and if HBsAg-positive, administer HBIG (no later than age 1 week).
   - If mother is HBsAg-negative, the birth dose can only be delayed with physician's order and mothers' negative HBsAg laboratory report documented in the infant's medical record.

   After the birth dose:
   - The HepB series should be completed with either monovalent HepB or a combination vaccine containing HepB. The second dose should be administered at age 1-2 months. The final dose should be administered at age ≥24 weeks. Infants born to HBsAg-positive mothers should be tested for HbsAg and antibody to HBsAg after completion of ≥3 doses of a licensed HepB series, at age 9-18 months (generally at the next well-child visit).

   4-month dose:
   - It is permissible to administer 4 doses of HepB when combination vaccines are administered after the birth dose. If monovalent HepB is used for doses after the birth dose, a dose at age 4 months is not needed.

2. **Rotavirus vaccine (Rota).** *(Minimum age: 6 weeks)*
   - Administer the first dose at age 6-12 weeks. Do not start the series later than age 12 weeks.
   - Administer the final dose in the series by age 32 weeks. Do not administer a dose later than age 32 weeks.
   - Data on safety and efficacy outside of these age ranges are insufficient.

3. **Diphtheria and tetanus toxoids and acellular pertussis vaccine (DTaP).** *(Minimum age: 6 weeks)*
   - The fourth dose of DTaP may be administered as early as age 12 months, provided 6 months have elapsed since the third dose.
   - Administer the final dose in the series at age 4-6 years.

4. **Haemophilus influenzae type b conjugate vaccine (Hib).** *(Minimum age: 6 weeks)*
   - If PRP-OMP (PedvacHIB® or ComVax® [Merck]) is administered at ages 2 and 4 months, a dose at age 6 months is not required.
   - TriHiBit® (DTaP/Hib) combination products should not be used for primary immunizations but can be used as boosters following any Hib vaccine in children aged ≥12 months.

5. **Pneumococcal vaccine.** *(Minimum age: 6 weeks for pneumococcal conjugate vaccine [PCV]; 2 years for pneumococcal polysaccharide vaccine [PPV])*

   - Administer PCV at ages 24-59 months in certain high-risk groups. Administer PPV to children aged ≥2 years in certain high-risk groups. See *MMWR* 2000;49(No. RR-9): 1-35.

6. **Influenza vaccine.** *(Minimum age: 6 months for trivalent inactivated influenza vaccine [TIV]; 5 years for live, arrenuated influenza vaccine [LAIV])*
   - All children aged 6-59 months and close contacts of all children aged 0-59 months are recommended to receive influenza vaccine.
   - Influenza vaccine is recommended annually for children aged ≥59 months with certain risk factors, health-care workers, and other persons (including household members) in close contact with person in groups at high risk. See *MMWR* 2006;55(No. RR-10):1-41.
   - For healthy person aged 5-49 years, LAIV may be used as an alternative to TIV.
   - Children receiving TIV should receive 0.25 mL if aged 6-35 months or 0.5 mL if aged ≥3 years.
   - Children <9 years who are receiving influenza vaccine for the first time should receive 2 doses (separated by ≥4 weeks for TIV and ≥6 weeks for LAIV).

7. **Measles, mumps, and rbella vaccine (MMR).** *(Minimum age: 12 months)*
   - Administer the second dose of MMR at age 4-6 years. MMR may be administered before age 4-6 years, provided ≥4 weeks have elapsed since the first dose and both doses are administered at age ≥12 months.

8. **Varicella vaccine.** *(Minimum age: 12 months)*
   - Administer the second dose of varicella vaccine at age 4-6 years. Varicella vaccine may be administered before age 4-6 years, provided that ≥3 months have elapsed since the first dose and both doses are administered at age ≥12 months. If second dose was administered ≥28 days following the first dose, the second dose does not need to be repeated.

9. **Hepatitis A vaccine (HepA).** *(Minimum age: 12 months)*
   - HepA is recommended for all children aged 1 year (i.e., aged 12-23 months). The 2 doses in the series should be administered at least 6 months apart.
   - Children not fully vaccinated by age 2 years can be vaccinated at subsequent visits.
   - HepA is recommended for certain other groups of children, including in areas where vaccination programs target older children. See *MMWR* 2006;55(No. RR-7):1-23.

10. **Meningococcal polysaccharide vaccine (MPSV4).** *(Minimum age: 2 years)*
    - Administer MPSV4 to children aged 2-10 years with terminal complement deficiencies or anatomic or functional aspenia and certain other high-risk groups. See *MMWR* 2005;54(No. RR-7):1-21.

The Recommended Immunization Schedules for Persons Aged 0-18 Years are approved by the Advisory Committee on Immunization Practices (http://www.cdc.gov/nip/acip), the American Academy of Pediatrics (http://www.aap.org), and the American Academy of Family Physicians (http://www.aafp.org).

FIGURE 2: Recommended Immunization schedule for persons aged 7-18 years — United States, 2007

Vaccine	7-10 years	11-12 YEARS	13-14 years	15 years	16-18 years
Tetanus, Diphtheria, Pertussis[1]	See footnote 1	Tdap	Tdap		
Human Papillomavirus[2]	See footnote 2	HPV (3 doses)	HPV series		
Meningococcal[3]	MPSV4	MCV4	MCV4[2]		
			MCV4		
Pneumococcal[4]	PPV				
Influenza[5]	Influenza (Yearly)				
Hepatitis A[6]	HepA Series				
Hepatitis B[7]	HepB Series				
Inactivated Poliovirus[8]	IPV Series				
Measles, Mumps, Rubella[9]	MMR Series				
Varicella[10]	Varecella Series				

Range of recommended ages

Catch-up immunization

Certain high-risk groups

This schedule indicates the recommended ages for routine administration of currently licensed childhood vaccines, as of December 1, 2006, for children aged 0-6 years. Additional information is available at http://www.cdc.gov/nip/recs/child-schedule.htm. Any dose not administered at the recommended age should be administered at any subsequent visit, when indicated and feasible. Additional vaccines may be licensed and recommended during the year. Licensed combination vaccines may be used whenever any components of the combination are indicated and other components of the vaccine are not contraindicated and if approved by the Food and Drug Administration for that dose of the series. Providers should consult the respective Advisory Committee on Immunization Practices statement for detailed recommendations. Clinically significant adverse events that follow immunization should be reported to the Vaccine Adverse Event Reporting System (VAERS). Guidance about how to obtain and complete a VAERS form is available at http://www.vaers.hhs.gov or by telephone, 800-822-7967.

1. **Tetanus and diphtheria toxoids and acellular pertussis vaccine (Tdap).** *(Minimum age: 10 years for BOOSTRIX® and 11 years for ADACEL™)*
   - Administer at age 11-12 years for those who have completed the recommended childhood DTP/DTaP vaccination series and have not received a tetanus and diphtheria toxoids vaccine (Td) booster dose.
   - Adolescents aged 13-18 years who missed the 11-12 year Td/Tdap booster dose should also receive a single dose of Tdap if they have completed the recommended childhood DTP/DTaP vaccination series.

2. **Human papillomavirus vaccine (HPV).** *(Minimum age: 9 years)*
   - Administer the first dose of the HPV vaccine to females at age 11-12 years.
   - Administer the second dose 2 months after the first dose and the third dose 6 months after the first dose.
   - Administer the HPV vaccine series to females at age 13-18 years if not previously vaccinated.

3. **Meningococcal vaccine.** *(Minimum age: 11 years for meningococcal conjugate vaccine [MCV4]; 2 years for meningococcal polysaccharide vaccine [MPSV4])*
   - Administer MCV4 at age 11-12 years and to previously unvaccinated adolescents at high school entry (at approximately age 15 years).
   - Administer MCV4 to previously unvaccinated college freshmen living in dormitories; MPSV4 is an acceptable alternative.
   - Vaccination against invasive meningococcal disease is recommended for children and adolescents aged ≥2 years with terminal complement deficiencies or aratomic or functional aspienia and certain other high-risk groups. See MMWR 2005;54(No. RR-7):1-21. Use MPSV4 for children aged 2-10 years and MCV4 or MPSV4 for older children.

4. **Pneumococcal polysaccharide vaccine (PPV).** *(Minimum age: 2 years)*
   - Administer for certain high-risk groups. See MMWR 1997;46(No. RR-8):1-24, and MMWR 2000;49(No. RR-9):1-35.

5. **Influenza vaccine.** *(Minimum age: 6 months for trivalent inactivated influenza vaccine [TIV], 5 years for live, attenuated influenza vaccine [LAIV])*
   - Influenza vaccine is recommended annually for persons with certain risk factors, health-care workers, and other persons (including household members) in close contact with person in groups at high risk. See MMWR 2006;55(No. RR-10):1-41.
   - For healthy person aged 5-49 years, LAIV may be used as an alternative to TIV.
   - Children aged <9 years who are receiving influenza vaccine for the first time should receive 2 doses (separated by ≥4 weeks for TIV and ≥6 weeks for LAIV).

6. **Hepatitis A vaccine (HepA).** *(Minimum age: 12 months)*
   - The 2 doses in the series should be administered at least 6 months apart.
   - HepA is recommended for certain other groups of children, including in areas where vaccination programs target older children. See MMWR 2006;55(No. RR-7):1-23.

7. **Hepatitis B vaccine (HepB).** *(Minimum age: birth)*
   - Administer the 3-dose series to those who were not previously vaccinated.
   - A 2-dose series of Recombivax HB® is licensed for children ages 11-15 years.

8. **Inactivated poliovirus vaccine (IPV).** *(Minimum age: 6 weeks)*
   - For children who received an all-IPV or all-oral poliovirus (OPV) series, a fourth dose is not necessary if the third dose was administered at age ≥4 years.
   - If both OPV and IPV were administered as part of a series, a total of 4 doses should be administered, regardless of the child's current age.

9. **Measles, mumps, and rubella vaccine (MMR).** *(Minimum age: 12 months)*
   - If not previously vaccinated, administer 2 doses of MMR during any visit, with ≥4 weeks between the doses.

10. **Varicella vaccine.** *(Minimum age: 12 months)*
    - Administer 2 doses of varicella vaccine to persons without evidence of immunity.
    - Administer 2 doses of varicella vaccine to person aged ≤13 years at least 3 months apart. Do not repeat the second dose, if administered ≥28 days after the first dose.
    - Administer 2 doses of varicella vaccine to persons aged ≥13 years at least 4 weeks apart.

The Recommended Immunization Schedules for Persons Aged 0-18 Years are approved by the Advisory Committee on Immunization Practices (http://www.cdc.gov/nip/acip), the American Academy of Pediatrics (http://www.aap.org), and the American Academy of Family Physicians (http://www.aafp.org).

Hepatitis B

What is Hepatitis B?

Hepatitis B virus (HBV) is an infection that affects the liver. The hepatitis B vaccine is different from other vaccines in that the illness is not considered a common childhood disease nor is it contagious. According to the CDC, "Although [the hepatitis B virus] is present in moderate concentrations in saliva, it's not transmitted commonly by casual contact."

The rates for hepatitis B are lower in the United States and Europe compared to other parts of the world. In the Far East and Africa, hepatitis B affects 5 to 20 percent of the population, while the lowest rates are found in the United States and Western Europe (0.1 to 0.5 percent). It is most common in adults ages 20 to 39; otherwise, it is uncommon in the general population in the United States.

The demographics of this illness make it an unusual choice for a mandated vaccine for every child. Cases of hepatitis B are more common in those who are sexually promiscuous or use IV drugs (60 to 80 percent of drug users have evidence of exposure), and can be contracted from blood transfusions or from occupational exposure, a particular risk for hospital workers. It is spread through infected bodily fluids such as blood, semen, vaginal secretions, and saliva, making it possible for an infected mother to transmit HBV to her baby during birth. It is for this reason that pregnant women are routinely screened for hepatitis B. Among children, it is those born to infected mothers who are at highest risk for developing chronic hepatitis B infections.

Symptoms of Hepatitis B

Initially, an infected person may have no signs of the disease. In fact, 30 percent of people show no signs or symptoms of the disease, and symptoms in children are less common than in adults. When symptoms do manifest, they may resemble a general flu-like feeling, including weakness, loss of appetite, nausea, headache, fatigue, diarrhea, joint pain, and pain in the right upper abdomen. Jaundice, including yellowing of the eyes, dark urine, and light-colored stools are also possible signs of HBV. Ninety-five percent of people who acquire hepatitis B recover fully and acquire lifelong immunity. The remaining 5 percent can become chronic carriers, and approximately 1.5 percent of these are in danger of developing liver disease.

Complications of Hepatitis B

Babies born to mothers with hepatitis B are at risk for contracting the disease at birth, with a 90 percent risk of chronic infection. Otherwise, hepatitis B is not considered a childhood disease. Five to 10 percent of cases become chronic, and may lead to liver damage, liver cancer, and liver failure (1 to 3 percent). Currently the CDC is promoting the vaccine as the first anti-cancer vaccine. According to the CDC, "Hepatitis B vaccine prevents hepatitis B disease and its serious consequences like hepatocellular carcinoma (liver cancer). Therefore, this is the first anti-cancer vaccine."

How Common Is Hepatitis B?

In general, the number of cases of hepatitis B is decreasing because of increased awareness of the disease and safer sexual and drug practices. In 1996, there were 10,637 cases of hepatitis B reported in the United States with 279 cases reported in children under the age of 14.

Treatment of Hepatitis B

HBV is diagnosed through a blood test. Medications such as interferon are often prescribed, though their efficacy is limited. Some adults with hepatitis B have begun to use complementary and alternative medicine to help boost their constitution, immune system, and liver. These include such modalities as homeopathy, acupuncture, herbal medicine, and naturopathic medicine.

Hepatitis B Vaccine (Recombivax HB)

In the past the vaccine was recommended for newborns who mothers tested positive for hepatitis B. Nowadays, the recommended immunization schedule is for three doses to be given: initially at birth, 1 to 2 months, and 6 to 18 months. Nevertheless, in 1991, the Advisory Committee on Immunization Practices (ACIP) of the Centers for Disease Control and Prevention (CDC) recommended that all infants be given the first dose of hepatitis B vaccine at birth before being discharged from the hospital newborn nursery.

The hepatitis B vaccine is known to contain mercury. The vaccine should target infants born to infected mothers, as these children are at highest risk for developing chronic hepatitis B infections. It is for this reason that pregnant women are routinely screened for hepatitis B.

Risks of the Vaccine

There are many medical articles linking the hepatitis B vaccine to demyelinating and autoimmune diseases such as multiple sclerosis. In addition, according to Burton A. Waisbren, M.D., a cell biologist and infectious disease specialist, "there are an increasing number of reports in the refereed medical literature about demyelinizing diseases occurring after an individual has received the hepatitis B vaccination...."

In addition, the hepatitis B vaccine has been linked to Guillain-Barré Syndrome, diabetes, and arthritis. At the American Diabetes Association annual meeting in 2000, Dr. Paolo Pozzili, professor of pediatrics at the University of Rome, presented research suggesting the hepatitis B vaccine is associated with an increase of type 1 diabetes in children. This included children who have close family members with type 1 diabetes. According to the Vaccine Adverse Event Reporting Systems (VAERS) there have been reports of sudden infant death syndrome (SIDS) in babies under one month old following the vaccine. Since 1990, more than 16,000 reported health problems stemming from the hepatitis B vaccine have been reported. Because it is estimated that only 10 percent of doctors report problems following a vaccination generally, the incidence of complications from vaccines like HBV could be in fact much higher.

Some patients have also reported becoming positive for hepatitis B on routine blood tests results following a hepatitis B vaccine. In addition, antibody levels from the vaccine probably decrease by the time a vaccinated child has reached the teen years when exposure to hepatitis B is more likely. Therefore, the vaccine may not in fact be as effective as it is thought to be. The FDA licensed the current hepatitis B vaccine despite a lack of adequate long-term follow-up studies; thy primarily used data that studied children for only 4 to 5 days following the vaccine.

The former hepatitis B vaccine was manufactured from human blood taken from chronic hepatitis B carriers. The current vaccine is a genetically engineered DNA recombinant called Recombivax HB. Recombinant DNA is manufactured when DNA (the genetic material) from one organism is transferred and inserted into another. Although there appear to be many advantages to using recombinant DNA, it has not been in use long enough to tell what the long-term effects will be.

Comments

It is reasonable to consider the hepatitis B vaccine if an infant is at high risk. However, because hepatitis B is not a common childhood illness, not highly contagious, and not in epidemic form in the United States (except among high-risk groups like IV drug addicts), it is unreasonable to mandate this vaccination, which has been associated with a multitude of adverse effects, for all children regardless of their risk. In addition, the "anti-cancer" campaign can be misleading to the public because that people in general are fearful of cancer, and may not know all facts and fallacies of this disease and the vaccine.

Rotavirus

What is Rotavirus?

Rotavirus is a common cause of acute diarrhea in children from three months to two years old. It is very easily spread. Once a child has had rotavirus, he or she may have repeat infections, although subsequent bouts tend to be less severe than the original. The incubation period is 2 days, and in uncomplicated cases the illness can last from 3 to 8 days. It is more common in the winter and spring.

Symptoms of Rotavirus

Rotavirus, also known as acute viral gastroenteritis, often begins with nausea, vomiting, and fever followed by severe watery diarrhea. Loss of appetite, cramps, and bloating are also common. There is no specific conventional treatment for it other than supportive therapy such as fluids and rest.

How Common Is Rotavirus?

Rotavirus is the leading cause of diarrhea worldwide. Nearly all American children have had the rotavirus infection by the age of five.

Complications of Rotavirus

Complications from severe diarrhea can lead to dehydration, which can be a serious health concern, especially in infants and young children. In the United States, rotavirus is responsible for approximately 55,000 hospitalizations a year, and 20 to 60 deaths. Over half a million children die from acute diarrhea illnesses in developing countries around the world annually.

Rotavirus Vaccine (RotaTeq)

The U.S. Food and Drug Administration approved a live virus vaccine (Rotashield) using a genetic human-monkey strain of rotavirus to be given to children beginning in 1998. However, due to severe side effects following the vaccine, including vomiting, diarrhea, and bowel obstruction (intussusception), the vaccine was removed from the market in 1999.

Currently a new live oral vaccine, RotaTeq, has been approved for prevention of rotavirus. It is in liquid form and given by mouth. The CDC recommendations have approved the vaccine to be given to infants in three doses, at 2, 4, and 6 months or before 32 weeks old. RotaTeq is human-bovine based and does not contain mercury (thimerosal).

Risks of the Vaccine

As this vaccine is newly marketed, substantial information on the effects of this vaccine is lacking. The FDA has alerted practitioners about reports that the RotaTeq vaccine has also been linked to intussusception, a twisting of the bowel that can lead to obstruction, like its predecessor, Rotashield. According to the FDA, "of the reported 28 cases of intussusception, the number that may have been caused by the vaccine, or occurred by coincidence, is unknown." During the clinical trials, 2.4 percent suffered serious adverse effects; these included bronchiolitis, gastroenteritis, pneumonia, fever, and urinary tract infections.

Comments

In the United States, rotavirus is a common childhood illness that usually resolves with supportive therapy. With serious side effects reported during the clinical trials of Rotateq, the jury is still out with this new vaccine which has also been linked to severe bowel obstruction, like its predecessor Rotashield.

Diphtheria, Tetanus, and Pertussis (DTaP)

The DTaP (diphtheria, tetanus, and acellular pertussis) is a three-in-one *trivalent* shot. Although many parents prefer separated shots, it is not possible to isolate the pertussis (whooping cough); it can only be given as a trivalent vaccine However, tetanus is available either singularly or with diphtheria. The DTaP series begins at 2 months of age. There are five doses given at 2 months, 4 months, 6 months, 15 to 18 months, and 4 to 6 years old.

Diphtheria
What is Diphtheria?

Diphtheria is a bacterial infection caused by *Corynebacterium diphtheriae* that produces toxins in the bloodstream. It is contagious and spreads through close contact with an infected person who may be a carrier without symptoms. The incubation period for diphtheria is 2 to 5 days.

Symptoms of Diphtheria

Diphtheria starts with sore throat symptoms as well as fever, chills, headache, cough, swollen glands, and runny nose. A membrane forms in the throat and tonsils making it difficult to swallow and sometimes interferes with breathing. Although diphtheria can affect the skin, it most often remains in the respiratory tract.

Complications of Diphtheria

Complications occur from the toxins produced that circulate through the body, causing damage to the heart muscle (myocarditis), kidney damage, neuritis, and temporary paralysis of limbs and muscles. The membrane in the back of the throat can also block the airways causing breathing difficulties.

How Common Is Diphtheria?

Diphtheria can be found in many places throughout the world, but is more common in poor and densely populated areas. In the United States, Native Americans generally have higher rates of diphtheria infection than Whites; this is likely owing to socioeconomic status and poorer living conditions. Outbreaks occur throughout the world, including in vaccinated communities.

Before the diphtheria vaccine was introduced in the 1940s, the severity and death rate in the United States had begun to decrease. With widespread vaccinations, the disease has been virtually eradicated: In the 1940s, 18,000 cases were reported each year; that number has now dropped to less than five cases a year. From 1980 to 2000 only 10 percent of diphtheria cases in the United States occurred in children less than 5 years old. As the incidence in infants has decreased, however, a higher proportion of cases were found among older persons, due either to a waning immunization or no immunization at all, and among individuals with weakened immune systems. The overall fatality rate for diphtheria is 5 to 10 percent.

Treatment for Diphtheria

People infected with diphtheria are hospitalized and given an antitoxin, antibiotics, and supportive therapies. With early treatment, complete recovery is expected with no side effects. Close contacts are treated with preventive antibiotics and updated shots.

The Diphtheria Vaccine

The diphtheria vaccine, as noted above, is usually given in combination with pertussis and tetanus as the DTaP shot. In addition, there are two types of diphtheria vaccine that are administered with just the tetanus shot: the DT, the pediatric vaccine, and Td, for older children and adults. DT is available for children who cannot receive the pertussis shot, and it contains 3 to 5 times more diphtheria toxoid than the Td adult dose. Oddly, the more concentrated pediatric DT vaccine is not used in adults and children over age seven because of possible side effects, according to vaccine expert Dr. Sherri Tenpenny. The Td is used instead as the booster. The CDC recommends that adults get the boosters of tetanus-diphtheria (Td) vaccine every 10 years.

Risks of the Vaccine

Since the diphtheria vaccination is given either in combination with pertussis and tetanus, or with the tetanus, side effects cannot be isolated. Adverse reactions to diphtheria and tetanus toxoid include local reaction of pain, swelling, and redness at the site of the injection; less common are fever and severe systemic complications.

There is evidence that outbreaks of diphtheria have occurred around the world following vaccination. Severe allergic reactions known as the Arthus type III hypersensitivity reaction have been known to occur following repeated diphtheria and tetanus vaccines. The DT and Td are often still manufactured with thimerosal (mercury).

Comments

Diphtheria is one of the vaccines whose risks and benefits become eclipsed by the more well-known components of tetanus and pertussis, with which it is usually given. Safety questions are raised about why the pediatric dose for smaller children is larger than the adult dose. Because diphtheria is rare in the United States and early treatment results in complete recovery, it is not usually one of utmost concern in parents who choose a selected shot schedule.

Tetanus
What Is Tetanus?

Tetanus, known as lockjaw, is caused by the *Clostridium tetani* bacterium, which produces a neurotoxin that is released causing severe symptoms in the muscles and nerves. Unlike most childhood illnesses, tetanus is not a contagious disease.

Tetanus is found in the soil in spores and enters the body through deep puncture wounds such as through stepping on a rusty nail. It can also occur in burns, frostbite, or other major injuries. The incubation period for tetanus is usually 3 to 21 days, with most symptoms beginning around the eighth day. Tetanus can also occur in newborns from an infected umbilical stump and unsanitary birth conditions, with symptoms starting within the first 2 weeks of life.

Symptoms of Tetanus

There are four known types of tetanus: local, cephalic, neonatal, and generalized, the latter of which affects all the skeletal muscles and is the most common as well as the most severe. Tetanus starts with difficulty swallowing, painful spasms, and tightening in the jaw (also called lockjaw). These symptoms can lead to severe muscle contractions and spasms in the neck, belly, back, and thighs. Symptoms can last 3 to 4 weeks, and full recovery can take several months.

Complications of Tetanus

Complications associated with tetanus include pneumonia, fractures (from severe muscle spasms), and brain damage. Extreme spasm of the breathing muscles can lead to death. In newborns, tetanus that can occur from an infected umbilical cord presents with severe spasms, poor feeding and rigidity. In general, the mortality rate is 30 percent, and is more common in adults over 60 years old. Occurring mostly in underdeveloped countries due to unhygienic conditions, neonatal tetanus affects infants up to 10 days old and has a higher mortality rate of 70 percent.

How Common Is Tetanus?

Tetanus is more common in developing countries of Africa, Asia, and South America. In 2002, 25 cases were reported in the United States and three deaths, most of them in adults. From 1980 to 2002 over 90 percent of cases were reported in adults over the age of 40; many were vaccinated. Recently, tetanus is on the rise in younger age groups, due mainly to the use of "dirty" needles among IV drug abusers, tattoos, and body piercing. More cases are diagnosed in the summer and wet season.

We have been ingrained with the notion that nearly any wound can cause tetanus. Imagine my surprise when I took my son Quentin to the emergency room in Switzerland for sutures for a superficial facial cut, and his tetanus immunization history was not even requested.

While tetanus exists everywhere, it is present in higher concentration in manure and on farms. In addition to stepping on a rusty nail, a person can contract tetanus from gangrene, burns, crush injuries, frostbite, and deep or particularly dirty wounds. Tetanus is a major risk with IV drug users who reuse or share infected needles. In the past, there were cases of tetanus in newborns who were born in unsanitary conditions or who suffered from serious infections of the umbilical stump. Fortunately, both are rare due to improved sanitation in childbirth and cord-care hygiene.

Treatment of Tetanus

Tetanus is treated in the hospital with an antitoxin, antibiotics, and sedation. The wound may require surgical cleaning. Supportive measures include bed rest in a quiet dark environment. Tetanus is diagnosed based on clinical symptoms, as there are no confirmatory lab tests.

Tetanus Vaccine

The vaccine is made from the tetanus toxoid, which is a deadly poison. In the preparation, it must be significantly diluted and weakened in order to avoid severe reactions. Many question whether the vaccine is even effective. According to researcher Dr. Viera Scheibner, author of *Vaccination, 100 Years of Orthodox Research Shows That Vaccines Represent a Medical Assault on the Immune System*, a person who gets the illness tetanus does not develop an immunity to it, and 60 percent of people who contract tetanus have been fully vaccinated; the body, apparently, cannot build an immunity against poisons. Getting a tetanus shot every 10 years as recommended to assure protection may not provide adequate antibody levels against tetanus.

The vaccine is given as the tetanus toxoid in combination with DTaP and DT and singularly as tetanus toxoid (TT). The DTaP is given at 2, 4, 6, 15 to 18 months, and 4 to 6 years. The DT is the vaccine for young children who do not receive the pertussis vaccine either because it is contraindicated (i.e. history of seizures or previous reaction) or by choice. The Td, (for adults and children 7 years old and older) is given at 11 to 12 years old age if it has been 5 years since the last dose, with a Td booster shot given every 10 years. The DT, Td, and TT are often still manufactured with thimerosal (mercury).

An alternative to the vaccine series is the Tetanus-Immune globulin (TIG) shot, which can be given within 72 hours following a serious injury. The TIG shot is indicated if there is a history of reactions to the Td shot. It can be given to a patient who has never received a tetanus shot or whose immunization status is not known, and is meant to be given to children 7 years and older. It contains the tetanus toxin antibodies from a large group of donors who had been vaccinated. It provides protective levels for the injury via passive immunization: the body does not develop its own antibodies. Often at the same time, patients are given the Td (or DT pediatric) shot. With the TIG injection there is the possibility of viral or bacterial contamination; however, since 1985 it has been screened for HIV and hepatitis.

Risks of the Vaccine

Adverse reactions to the diphtheria and tetanus toxoid vaccine include pain, swelling, and redness at the site of the injection; less common are fever and severe systemic complications. Additional risks include incidence of tetanus, Guillain-Barré Syndrome, and arthritis. Allergic reactions occur when people have been sensitized from having received repeated tetanus shots. Known as the Arthus type III hypersensitivity reaction, it is a severe reaction at the site of the shot that leads to a local tissue necrosis (death) and vasculitis within hours of giving the shot. Arthus reaction may also occur from diphtheria toxoid.

Comments

An ounce of prevention is worth a pound of cure, and according to the *Journal of the American Medical Association*, "Good wound care is probably the single most important factor in the prevention of tetanus in fresh wounds." Although many parents are concerned about tetanus in their children, historically the most common type in children is in newborns (less than one month old) which would not even be covered by the standard schedule which typically begins at 2 months of age. Because it is not a contagious illness and precautions can be taken after an injury or wound, parents who have chosen not to vaccinate their children have the option of giving the TIG passive immunity following an injury for protection.

Pertussis (Whooping Cough)
What Is Pertussis?

Pertussis (whooping cough, named after the characteristic "whoop" sound heard during cough attacks) is a contagious illness caused by the *Bordatella pertussis* bacterium. In the United States it used to be a common childhood illness known as the 100-day cough. The bacteria spreads easily from contact with an infected child or adult in the first 2 to 3 weeks of the infection, usually before the illness is properly diagnosed.

Symptoms of Pertussis

The incubation period is commonly 5 to 10 days, but can be up to 21 days. Like many illnesses, pertussis starts with a cold-like stage (the most contagious phase) with familiar symptoms such as a runny nose, sneezing, low-grade fever, and mild cough. Within 1 to 2 weeks, the child begins to experience worsening of the cough, which can last from 1 to 6 weeks (the coughing fit stage). This develops into coughing spells that come in fits of rapid coughs followed by the characteristic long inspiration with a crowing sound or high-pitched whoop. Choking, gagging, or vomiting while coughing may be triggered by the thick mucus build up in the lungs. In more severe cases, a child may turn blue in the face; this is known as cyanosis. Although the child may be exhausted immediately following a coughing spell, he often appears and acts normal in between coughing fits. From beginning to end, the stages of whooping cough can last from weeks to a few months.

Having whooping cough does not provide lifelong immunity. Adolescents and adults who have previously had the infection in childhood may have milder forms of whooping cough, which may go undetected and diagnosed as a bronchitis or a simple cough. Pertussis is also a common cause of prolonged cough in adults. Often these cases are considered a source of infection to children.

Complications of Pertussis

The most common complication associated with whooping cough is pneumonia, which occurs in 5 percent of reported cases. The bacteria can also lead to ear infections, dehydration, convulsions, and, in rare instances, brain damage or death. Pertussis poses the greatest risk to infants (especially under 6 months of age) and small children, due to the small size of their air passages.

How Common Is Pertussis?

The Centers for Disease Control and Prevention (CDC) reports that the incidence of whooping cough has decreased 98 percent since the inception of the vaccine. In the holistic medical community, it is generally felt that pertussis is less severe now than in the past due to improvements in sanitation, nutrition, and education, and because of more sophisticated medical treatments for complications. In the United States, approximately 10,000 cases were reported in 2003, with outbreaks occurring every 3 to 4 years. Approximately half of whooping cough cases occur in children less than 5 years old; 13 children died of pertussis in the United States in 2003. As a common cause of persistent cough in adults, pertussis accounts for more than 17 percent of all coughs.

The rate of pertussis, however, has increased steadily since the 1980s. It is estimated that only one-third of pertussis cases in the United States are actually reported. Overall, adolescents and adults have seen increases in whooping cough, most likely attributable to their immunity waning in the years following the vaccine.

Treatment of Pertussis

See your pediatrician if you suspect your child has whooping cough. It will usually last approximately 6 weeks no matter what the treatment. Because pertussis is contagious, infected persons should avoid contact with others.

Standard treatment includes the general support of rest and liquids. Your doctor will prescribe an antibiotic such as erythromycin as it is felt that the antibiotic renders your child less contagious. While it remains questionable whether the antibiotic changes the course of the illness, people are generally no longer considered contagious after the fifth day on antibiotics. There are also many homeopathic and natural remedies available for pertussis.

The Pertussis Vaccine

The pertussis vaccine is given as a part of the DTaP (diphtheria, tetanus, and acellular pertussis) series beginning at 2 months of age. There are five doses given at 2, 4, 6, 15 to 18 months, and 4 to 6 years. The severe complications caused by the original whole-cell pertussis vaccine led to the development of the acellular pertussis (aP) vaccine, while the publicity surrounding the original pertussis vaccine complications is to a large extent responsible for the current public awareness about vaccine injuries.

Risks of the Vaccine

Complications from the original pertussis vaccine are well-documented and include local swelling, fever, high-pitched screaming, convulsions, mental retardation, disabilities, and death. Reactions to acellular form of the pertussis vaccine are milder compared to the whole-cell vaccine; however, severe reactions to the acellular vaccine also occur, including encephalitis and death.

The DTaP is only given to children less than 7 years of age as it is not licensed in older children. Protection lasts approximately 5 to 10 years. Recently the Tdap was introduced as the trivalent vaccine suggested for adolescents and adults who have waning immunity from pertussis. The current suggested age of immunization is 11 to 12 years old. In this formulation, the concentration of diphtheria is reduced to prevent adverse sensitivity reactions that could be caused by accumulation of antigen from successive doses of diphtheria. The pertussis vaccine should not be given to children who have a history of convulsions, brain disorder, or abnormal development. Some of my families have refused the pertussis shot if there is a family history of seizures.

Comments
Due to increased standards of living in our country, whooping cough, whose number of cases is vastly underreported, is not the grave disease that it used to be and is much more manageable with less incidence of complications and death. For many new parents, though, pertussis remains a concern and is one of the more common priority vaccines given in baby's first year. Although the newer version of the vaccine (DTaP) contains less pertussis toxin and is associated with less mild reactions, severe problems and death have been reported. Because of waning immunity, adolescents and adults who were vaccinated as children remain vulnerable to whooping cough and can become carriers.

Haemophilus Influenza Type B (Hib)
What Is Hib?
Haemophilus influenzae type b (Hib) meningitis is a bacterial infection. It received its name because it was believed to be the cause of the influenza virus in the late 1800s (it isn't). The haemophilus influenza bacteria normally lives dormant in the mouth and nose of most people and is responsible for many mild ear, nose, and throat infections. On rare occasions, the type b strain becomes more invasive, leading to more severe infections, including meningitis. Hib is contagious even among carriers who show no signs of the disease, and spreads through person-to-person contact, including coughing, sneezing, and other exchanges of respiratory droplets and secretions from the mouth.

In the past, Hib was not a common infection in newborns and adults. From 1946 to 1986, however, the frequency and severity of Hib increased at a fourfold rate. Researchers believe this may be due to bacterial resistance caused by excessive use of antibiotics. Some cases of sinus and ear infections are also caused by Hib. Hib infections occur most often from September to December and from March to May. Before the vaccine was introduced, it accounted for approximately 50 percent of meningitis cases. The incubation period is not known. The risk factors include severely weakened immune systems (immune compromised), overcrowded living spaces, daycare, lower socioeconomic status, and less educated families.

Children less than 6 months old are considered to be protected by maternal antibodies. Breastfeeding offers protection for children from meningitis. In fact the longer a child is breastfed, the less is the risk of meningitis. This protection has been documented by Swedish researchers to last up to 5 to 10 years following weaning.

Symptoms of Hib
Hib is responsible for many mild ear, nose, and throat infections, which have symptoms similar to a cold. Hib meningitis, which is a more severe infection, usually follows a cold-like illness. The symptoms in young children include fussiness, nausea, vomiting, and poor feeding, often accompanied by high fever. The commonly associated symptoms of meningitis, which include neck and back stiffness, sensitivity to light, sleepiness, and a severe headache, may be more difficult to detect in infants or may even be absent. Other serious signs are mental confusion, shock, and coma. In severe cases of Hib, a child can die within several hours.

Complications of Hib
Meningitis is the most common and severe complication of Hib infection. In general, meningitis is a serious infection that can affect both children and adults in viral and bacterial forms. Meningitis is an infection of the covering

around the brain (meninges) and in the spinal cord. While viral meningitis is less severe and often requires no treatment, bacterial meningitis constitutes a serious health threat, accounting for 80 percent of infections including *Neisseria meningitidis* (meningococcus), *Haemophilus influenzae* type b, and *Streptococcus pneumoniae* (pneumococcus). In recent years, *Haemophilus influenzae* type b was the most common cause of bacterial meningitis in the United States.

Complications from bacterial meningitis can include pneumonia, arthritis, pericarditis (infection around the heart), hearing loss, seizures, brain damage and learning disabilities in approximately 15 to 30 percent of cases, with a mortality rate of 2 to 5 percent.

How Common Is Hib?

The increase of Hib in recent decades prompted the development of the Hib vaccine. Since the introduction of the vaccine there has been a 95 percent reduction in the disease. Before the vaccine, Hib was the most common cause of bacterial meningitis in babies and young children. Nearly all cases of Hib occur in children under 5 years of age. In 1984, there were 20,000 cases of Hib meningitis recorded, the highest in one year. From 1996 to 2000 there were approximately 68 cases a year. By 2002, only 34 cases of Hib disease were confirmed.

Treatment of Hib

The response to early treatment of Hib is favorable. The Hib diagnosis is made from a spinal tap (lumbar puncture) to examine the fluid in the spinal canal (cerebrospinal fluid). Treatment usually requires hospitalization, accompanied by antibiotics and supportive therapies. Some strains are beginning to be resistant to particular antibiotics. Oxygen, blood transfusion, and other therapies may be required. Household contacts are treated preventively with antibiotics. The illness may provide permanent immunity; however, this is not the case in children who are immune compromised or who are younger than 2 years old.

The Hib Vaccine

The Hib vaccine was first introduced in 1985, but was discontinued when it was discovered to result in increased susceptibility to the illness in children over 18 months in the first week following the vaccine. It was also considered not to be effective in children younger than 18 months old. Currently, a newer and more effective conjugate Hib vaccine is in wide use. The CDC recommends the following schedule for the Hib vaccine: 2, 4, 6, and 12 to 15 months. It may be given simultaneously with the hepatitis B vaccine; the combined vaccine is called the Combivax.

Risks of the Vaccine

Reactions to Hib vaccine include fever, irritability, prolonged crying, diarrhea, vomiting convulsions, shock, collapse, Hib meningitis, and Guillain-Barré Syndrome. Up to 30 percent of children experience pain, redness, or swelling around the injection site. It is difficult to determine the reaction caused by the Hib vaccine because it is usually given in the same time schedule as the DTaP and other shots. Research into potential reactions to the Hib vaccine is still lacking.

Comments

Hib meningitis is a serious illness, and one of the more important vaccines that many of my patients consider during baby's first year. Mothers should consider breastfeeding beyond one year because of its overall health benefits and its association with lower incidence of Hib meningitis.

Pneumococcal

What Is Pneumococcal?

Streptococcus pneumonia (pneumococcus) is a bacterium that is found in the nose and throat of most children and adults. Not to be confused with group A streptococcus (which causes strep throat), pneumococcus occasionally leads to an invasive infection causing ear and sinus infections or, in more severe cases, pneumonia, meningitis, and blood infection. In fact, it is considered a common cause of fevers (without other symptoms) in children under 2 years old. There are 90 types of pneumococcal bacteria known, and 30 percent are already resistant to antibiotics.

Symptoms of Pneumococcal

Symptoms of pneumococcal disease include general discomfort and fever. Pneumococcal ear infections are painful and may fill with pus, which can lead to perforated eardrum with drainage. If there is pneumonia, symptoms will progress with chills, cough, blood-tinged sputum, difficult rapid breathing, and chest pain. Symptoms of meningitis are different and include fussiness, high fever, lack of appetite, vomiting, headache, and neck stiffness.

Complications of Pneumococcal

Pneumococcal infections affect young children more often than older children and adults.

Pneumococcus is considered a common cause of fever and middle ear and sinus infections. More rare but more serious complications include pneumonia, meningitis, and bacteremia (infections in the blood). Those at high risk of developing severe invasive infection include children with weakened immune systems (such as those on chemotherapy), those with spleen and kidney diseases, children less than 2 years old, the elderly, children of Native American descent, African-American children, and children who spend a minimum of 4 hours a week in a daycare setting. Pneumococcal infection is more common in the winter and early spring. The mortality rate from pneu-mococcal meningitis infection is approximately 8 percent.

How Common Is Pneumococcal?

In the United States, there are approximately 280 cases a year of meningitis, 4,600 cases a year of bacteremia (blood poisoning), and 3.1 million ear infec-tions in children younger than 5 years old caused by pneumococcal infections. According to the CDC, pneumococcal infections cause approximately 100 deaths a year in the United States.

The Pneumococcal Vaccine (PCV7 or Prevnar)

The heptavalent pneumococcal conjugate vaccine (PCV7), also known as Prevnar, is given at 2, 3, and 6 months of age with a minimum of 6 weeks between doses. A fourth booster dose is recommended at 12 to 15 months. The vaccine contains only seven strains of pneumococcous (there are 90). Prevnar is given to infants and toddlers. Older children and adults may be given a different vaccine called the pneumococcal polysaccharide vaccine (PPV). This vaccine is approved for adults 65 years or older, and children older than 2 years who have chronic illness such as sickle-cell disease or dia-betes, or severely weakened immune system, from a condition such as cancer.

The PCV7 vaccine (Prevnar) was approved for use in 2000, despite the fact that many organizations, including the National Vaccine Information Center, question its effectiveness. According to Erdem Cantekin, Ph.D., pro-fessor of otolaryngology, University of Pittsburgh, an authority on otitis media (ear infection), "The alleged benefits for this new vaccine are greatly exaggerated and the risks are significant." The clinical trials of the vaccine were confusing, not scientifically acceptable, and not complete. Although it is recognized that pneumococcus causes disease, the role it plays and how it becomes a severe infection are unknown. Pneumococcus causes only about 25 percent of cases of ear infection.

Risks of the Vaccine

Side effects of the vaccine include local soreness and swelling, fever, irritability, and loss of appetite. In addition, children in one of the clinical trials who received the pneumococcal vaccine suffered high fevers, seizures, gastritis, asthma, and other reactions, including 12 deaths.

There have been no long-term studies evaluating the vaccine. According to the manufacturer's product insert, Prevnar may reduce the effectiveness of the Hib, pertussis, and polio vaccines if they are given as the same time.

Comments

Although the pneumococcus bacterium can cause serious infections on rare occasions, the vaccine only protects against 7 out of 90 strains of pneumococcus. In addition, there was a high incidence of adverse reactions during the clinical trials and there are no long-term studies yet on its effects. Given this information, many parents consider Prevnar a low-priority vaccine, in which the benefits of the vaccine may not outweigh the risks.

Polio

What is Polio?

Poliomyelitis (polio) is caused by a virus that spreads by contact with stool from an infected person; for example, eating food that has been handled by a carrier. Once a person is exposed, the virus enters through the mouth and lodges in the throat and intestines.

Symptoms of Polio

Surprisingly, over 95 percent of polio cases go unnoticed, or may present with mild complaints of sore throat, stomachache, nausea, headache, and flu-like symptoms. Most cases happen in children from 3 to 5 years old, and once infected there is lifelong immunity from the disease. Only 1 percent of polio cases become the classic paralytic polio in which the virus attacks the brain and spinal cord, and causes paralysis in different muscle groups. Regardless of symptoms, an infected person may increase rate of infections to others as the virus is shed in the stool for weeks. The incubation period for polio is commonly 3 to 20 days.

Complications of Polio

Paralysis is the most common and severe complication of polio. Paralysis most commonly affects the legs. In severe cases there can be paralysis of the muscles used for breathing and swallowing, which can be fatal. Half of the patients with paralytic polio fully recover within 3 to 6 months.

How Common Is Polio?

First described by a physician in the eighteenth century, polio outbreaks occurred frequently in the late 1800s. In the past, polio epidemics occurred mostly in the summer and fall. When I was growing up, I heard stories about my father and uncle having polio while away at summer camp, a not uncommon occurrence in the United States in the early to mid-twentieth century. Before the introduction of the vaccine in 1955, polio affected thousands of children every year.

In developing countries, most children are exposed to the polio virus as a result of poor sanitation and contaminated water supplies. Interestingly, this natural exposure to polio allows children to develop antibodies that boost their immunity to the disease. In the eighteenth and nineteenth centuries, the paralyzing form was relatively rare in our country, but as sanitation and water supplies improved, children became more susceptible to the virus, contributing to polio epidemics. In contrast to most other diseases, polio epidemics became more commonplace as sanitation improved.

In the United States, polio outbreaks prompted one of the largest nationwide vaccination programs in history, with millions of children receiving the newly developed inoculations. Like most people, I grew up with the notion that the polio vaccine was responsible for the dramatic decline in the disease. In 1962, however, Dr. Bernard Greenberg, head of the Department of Biostatistics for the University of North Carolina School of Public Health, testified at a congressional hearing that statistics were altered to give the public the impression that the vaccine had greatly altered polio rates. For instance, before 1955, cases of Guillain-Barré Syndrome were considered to be polio, which inflated the number of "polio" cases. After 1955, the criteria for diagnosis for paralytic polio changed, resulting in fewer polio diagnoses.

Currently, paralytic polio accounts for only 1 percent of all polio cases, and of these cases, 5 to 10 percent are fatal. Between 1980 and 1999 there were only 152 reported cases of paralytic polio, approximately 8 cases per year. Cases of polio in the United States are largely contracted from either the oral polio vaccine or from travel abroad. Outbreaks still occur throughout the world, including in vaccinated populations.

The Polio Vaccine (IPV)

Up until 2000, there were two polio vaccines: the inactivated polio virus or killed virus (IPV, developed by researcher Dr. Jonas Salk) given as a shot, or the oral polio virus (OPV, developed by Dr. Albert Sabin) taken by mouth. The OPV was discontinued in 2000 due to its links to cases of paralytic polio (known as VAPP, or vaccine-associated paralytic polio). Although the IPV is not associated with paralytic polio, it provides less protection than the OPV. Children now receive 4 doses of IPV (inactivated polio virus) at 2 months, 4 months, and 6 to 18 months, and receive a booster between 4 and 6 years of age. A child is considered to have 99 percent immunity after three doses (90 percent after two doses); however, the amount of time the protection lasts is uncertain.

The preparation of IPV is grown on monkey kidney cells. It is inactivated with formaldehyde and contains the antibiotics neomycin, streptomycin, and polymyxin B.

Risks of the Vaccine

The IPV can cause local swelling, pain, and redness, along with fever, fussiness, fatigue, and vomiting. With the discontinuation of the oral vaccine, vaccine-associated paralytic polio is no longer a risk. One of the more debilitating reactions associated with both vaccines is Guillain-Barré Syndrome (GBS), a condition that presents symptoms similar to polio.

From 1954 to 1963, the inactivated polio vaccine (IPV) was found to be contaminated with monkey virus (known as simian virus 40 or SV40), contracted from the monkey tissue used to grow the polio virus. Over 98 million Americans received the vaccination during that time period. Initially, the virus was not considered harmful to humans, but SV40 is now linked to brain, bone, and lymphatic cancers, including mesothelioma (tumors of the lining of lung and chest) and non-Hodgkins lymphoma. Although the IPV currently is not known to be contaminated with SV40, some children who were too young to receive the contaminated polio vaccines have suffered with similar cancers; it is unclear if there is a connection, or if this is simply coincidental.

Comments

Paralytic polio can be a crippling disease. This seems to be a good enough reason to justify getting inoculated against the disease. However, there is some evidence that the public has been misled to believe that the vaccine alone has been responsible for the decline in rates of polio. After considering both viewpoints, many of my patients choose to forego this vaccine altogether, citing its possible cancer connection with SV40.

Influenza

What Is Influenza?

Influenza gets its name from the Latin word "influence" because people believed that epidemics were due to influence from the stars. The flu is caused by various viruses that are classified into three types: A, B, and C. Type A is more common, can affect any age group, and is responsible for serious epidemic outbreaks that occur from November to March. Pandemics which affect multiple continents come from new strains of type A viruses, which can change every 2 to 3 years.

Outbreaks in the flu season also occur from type B viruses but are usually milder and affect children primarily (ages 5 to 14 years old). Type B is less changeable than type A, and immunity can last for many years.

Type C viruses are not associated with large outbreaks and are often confused with the common cold. Influenza type A contains different subtypes which infect humans, birds (avian flu), pigs, horses, and other animals. Types B and C are found in humans only, and have no subtypes. It is not common for human to get the flu from animals but occasional cross-species infection does occur; this is the concern about avian flu, which has infected several people in Asia and may mutate into a virus that spreads easily and causes more serious illness.

Symptoms of Influenza
Is it the flu or a cold? Symptoms of the flu are high fever, fatigue, headache, and body aches, and can include cold-like symptoms, such as a stuffy nose, sore throat, and cough. Common cold symptoms are more centered around the nose (rhinovirus) and associated with runny nose, congestion, sneezing, and low-grade fever, as well as sore throat and cough.

Complications of Influenza
Complications of the flu include secondary infections such as ear infections, sinus infections, bronchitis, and, more seriously, pneumonia. Pneumonia is a condition of the lungs and respiratory system caused by either infection or injury (such as from smoking). Symptoms of pneumonia are chest pain, fever, difficulty breathing, and cough. Children between 6 months and 5 years old, and people who have serious illnesses with compromised immune systems, as well as the elderly and pregnant women, are more susceptible to complications from the flu. There are over 35,000 deaths per year from the flu, mostly affecting people in these high-risk groups.

How Common Is Influenza?

According to the CDC, "influenza causes more hospitalizations and deaths among American children than any other vaccine-preventable disease; deriving accurate population-based estimates of disease impact is challenging." U.S. statistics report from 5 to 20 percent of the population has the flu each year, with 200,000 hospitalizations and 36,000 deaths from complications. This includes 20,000 children (under 5 years old) hospitalized for the flu annually.

Treatment of Influenza

The standard treatment of the flu includes general supportive measures such as rest, fluids, and over-the-counter medication for fever and muscle aches. Several antivirals are on the market for treatment and prevention of types A and B infections. One of these, Amantadine, is approved for treatment and prevention of uncomplicated type A virus in children who are 1 year old and older. However, in the 2006–7 flu season, the CDC recommended they not be used due to viral resistance. Side effects of Amantadine include difficulty sleeping, anxiety, loss of appetite, and nausea. Seizures can occur sometimes.

Homeopathy and herbal medicines can be helpful to alleviate symptoms and speed healing.

The Influenza Vaccine

The flu shot is an inactivated (killed) vaccine meant to prevent illnesses from types A and B flu viruses. Some of these preparations still contain mercury (thimerosal). Every year at the onset of the flu season, we are inundated in the media with information about flu prevention. It is implied that the flu shot could save many lives. The vaccine is reformulated to target the flu strains that are predicted to most likely cause a flu epidemic in that year. Parents of children 6 months and older are encouraged to get them a flu shot every autumn. The flu shot is recommended for women during pregnancy, even though it contains mercury.

In 2003, FluMist, a live weakened vaccine that can be given as a spray through the nostrils, was approved by the FDA. FluMist is not approved for children younger than 5 years old. In one study, FluMist was found to be approximately 86 percent effective against the flu. The flu shot, in contrast, ranges from 70 to 90 percent effective. These rates vary and are dependent on the year.

Risks of Vaccine

Reactions to the flu shot include flu-like symptoms such as localized soreness at the site of injection, fever, aches, and fatigue. More serious reactions include allergic reactions and Guillain-Barré Syndrome, an autoimmune illness. Because the vaccine is grown in egg culture, it is not recommended for people who have an allergy to eggs. According to Hugh Fudenberg, M.D., founder and Director of Research, Neuro Immuno Therapeutic Research Foundation, if an individual has had the flu shot consecutively at least five times, he or she increases the chance of getting Alzheimer's disease tenfold, probably because of the accumulation of aluminum and mercury in the brain.

Comments

Many families concerned about protection during the flu season often prefer natural and homeopathic medicines, because the flu shot contains mercury, and aluminum, and is grown in chicken eggs, to which many people are allergic. Given the fact that the shot contains thimerosal and other additives, it is ironic that it is suggested for pregnant women, despite the fact that they are also told to avoid fish with high heavy metal content.

Measles, Mumps, and Rubella (MMR)

The measles, mumps, and rubella (MMR) vaccines are commonly given as a three-in-one trivalent vaccine of live viruses at 1 year, with a second dose given between 4 and 6 years. The vaccine should not be given to children who are allergic to gelatin, neomycin, or eggs, since it is grown on chick embryo culture.

The MMR vaccine (along with the DTaP, hepatitis B, Hib, polio, and other vaccines) has been strongly linked to autism and pervasive developmental disorders. Although mainstream medicine believes that scientific evidence does not support this theory, many reports from parents have supported this. In 1998, Dr. Andrew Wakefield of the London Royal Free Hospital and his colleagues suggested that the MMR vaccine (especially the measles vaccine) may be the cause of an inflammatory bowel condition in children, which may be linked to autism. For this reason, many parents are cautious in giving the MMR and prefer that the shots be given separately.

Measles (Rubeola)
What Is Measles?

Measles used to be a common childhood virus before the vaccine. It occurred primarily in children ages 2 to 6 years, and almost every child had measles by the age of 15. Measles was such a common illness that people born before 1957 are probably immune to measles, as they probably had it in childhood or were exposed. It is extremely contagious and is spread through close contact with an infected person (4 days before to 4 days after rash onset) or through touching contaminated surfaces. The incubation period is approximately 10 to 12 days following exposure. A cyclical disease, measles outbreaks happen around the world every 2 to 3 years and more often in the late winter and early spring.

Symptoms of Measles

Most cases are mild, and begin with a high fever, then cold-like symptoms, including a runny nose, pinkeye, and a hacking cough. Within a few days, a red blotchy rash appears. It can be itchy with raised red bumps. Characteristically, Koplik spots, small white spots in the insides of the cheek, appear before the rash. The rash begins faintly behind the ears and within 24 hours becomes darker as it spreads to the face, head, neck, and arms (including hands). In 2 to 3 days, the rash reaches the legs, while the rash on the face correspondingly fades. With the onset of the rash, the child begins to feel better. Additional symptoms include sore throat, muscle pains, and light sensitivity. Most children who develop measles recover fully.

Complications of Measles

Occasionally there can be complications due to secondary infections. These may include diarrhea (in 8 percent of cases), ear infections (in 7 percent of cases), croup, and, in more severe cases, deafness, blindness, pneumonia, and encephalitis. The mortality rate is 1 in 1,000 cases.

How Common Is Measles?

In 1985, the government reported 80 percent of measles cases had been vaccinated. In 2002, 44 cases of measles were reported, which is substantially low, compared to 1941 when nearly 900,000 cases were reported. The vaccination program began in 1963, which has caused the occurrence of measles to shift to an older population. Outbreaks also occur in vaccinated populations.

Measles is still considered a severe illness in developing nations, where living conditions, sanitation, water supply, healthcare, and nutrition are considered inadequate. In past centuries, the mortality rate in the United States was higher than it is now. The current fatality rate is 1 to 2 out of 1,000 cases. Complications are more frequently seen in those with weakened immune systems, children with chronic disease, babies under 1 year old, and in adults.

After a child has had measles, he or she receives lifelong immunity from it. A mother who had measles as a child passes antibodies to her baby in utero, thus protecting her newborn for the first year of life. However, in the early 1990s there was a measles outbreak in the United States that included children who were younger than 1 year old, which was unusual. According to the CDC, this was due to mothers who had been vaccinated, but never had the natural disease. The CDC concluded that the protection from the vaccine decreases over time, and that the vaccinated mothers did not pass their natural maternal measles antibodies to their babies.

Treatment of Measles

Standard medicine has no treatment for measles. The symptoms of high fever and cold do not respond to antibiotics or cough medicine, though supportive treatment, such as rest and fluids, are helpful. Homeopathy, naturopathy, traditional Chinese medicine, and chiropractics have all been useful in the treatment of measles and in strengthening the body's natural ability to heal.

The Measles Vaccine

The vaccine is composed of a live attenuated virus. According to a CDC published article, "Maternal Antibodies Interfere with Measles Vaccination," some children who have received the measles vaccine or the MMR before 15 months of age may be in jeopardy of vaccine failure (in which the child fails to develop the desired immunity) because the immunity from the mother's antibodies counteracts or neutralizes the vaccine. This can occur, especially if the mother had measles as a child. According to the CDC, many of these children were vaccinated when 1 year to 14 months old.

Measles, mumps, and rubella (MMR) vaccines are given as a single shot of live viruses beginning at 1 year, with a second dose given at 4 to 6 years old. The vaccine is contraindicated in children who are allergic to eggs. When giving the measles shot alone, most parents follow the recommended schedule for the MMR vaccine with the first one given at around 15 months, and the second one before kindergarten. Because of possible interactions between the measles and mumps shots, separate the two by at least 6 months.

Risks of the Vaccine

Although most children receive the MMR in combination, there are adverse effects specific to each component. The measles vaccine, in particular, has been linked to colitis and various forms of inflammatory bowel disease. A study from the New York University School of Medicine involving autistic children found that 85 percent had severe intestinal inflammation, with evidence of measles virus on the biopsies. It is theorized that this inlammation may cause changes in the intestinal barrier, allowing the virus to enter the child's bloodstream and cause inflammation elsewhere, namely in the brain, thus contributing to the development of autism.

In general, mild side effects of the MMR vaccine include pain and swelling at the injection site, cold-like symptoms, fever, swollen glands, headache, dizziness, rash, nausea, and vomiting. More moderate adverse effects are convulsions, arthritis, thrombocytopenia (bleeding disorder), and Guillain-Barré. Very rarely there may be severe allergic life-threatening reactions, including deafness, comas, and permanent brain damage. The MMR vaccine has also been linked to autism.

Comments

Before the vaccination program was licensed in 1967, nearly every American child born before 1957 had measles. Most recovered without any serious consequences. With the possible link of the vaccine to inflammatory bowel disease and autism, many parents have questioned the use of the MMR vaccine, and if considering the measles vaccine at all, choose the single separated dose over the combined.

Mumps
What Is Mumps?

Mumps is a mild viral infection that used to be extremely common in children 5 to 14 years old. It is contagious and easily spread by person-to-person contact. Mumps is considered a mild illness in children, and more severe in teenagers and adults. It has an incubation period of 14 to 18 days. The infection is more common in late winter to spring.

Symptoms of Mumps

Twenty percent of mumps cases have no symptoms. Mumps begins with the common vague symptoms of fever, loss of appetite, headache, and fatigue. In up to 40 percent of cases, it leads within 24 hours to the characteristic painful swelling of the cheek between the ear and jaw (one or both sides), caused by inflammation of the salivary gland. The illness is usually over within one week, providing lifelong immunity.

Complications of Mumps

Complications are rare. They may include inflammation of the ovaries, testicles (more common in adolescent boys and men), and pancreas, deafness, encephalitis, and meningitis. Inflammation of the testicles (orchitis) occurs in 20 to 50 percent of post-pubertal males, though sterility is rare. Most of the cases of deafness (80 percent) are one-sided and occur in 1 out of 20,000 cases.

How Common Is Mumps?

In 2002, there were 270 cases reported, compared to 1968, when there was a peak of 152,209 cases. Mumps has a death rate of approximately 2 out of 10,000 cases. If you were born before 1957, you are considered immune to mumps.

Treatment of Mumps

Treatment for mumps infection includes bed rest, fluids, and a simple bland diet. Orange juice and other tart acidic juices should be avoided due to increased pain. Local compresses (warm or cold as tolerated) can be soothing. Other natural therapies, such as homeopathy, osteopathy, naturopathy, chiropractic, and Chinese medicine, are effective in aiding the healing process.

The Mumps Vaccine

The mumps vaccine is a live attenuated virus vaccine and was licensed in 1967. Measles, mumps, and rubella (MMR) vaccines are given as a single shot of live viruses beginning at 12 months, with a second dose given at 4 to 6 years old. The vaccine is contraindicated in children who are allergic to eggs. When administering the vaccine as a single shot, most parents roughly follow the recommended schedule giving the mumps vaccine during baby's second year, and another dose between 4 to 6 years old.

Risks of the Vaccine

The risks of the mumps vaccine as a single shot include meningitis and diabetes mellitus, as it can affect the pancreatic gland. The incidence of juvenile onset diabetes has greatly increased in recent years, and it has been suggested that the mumps vaccinations may contribute to this. Because young children are being vaccinated, mumps, which is more serious in adults, is becoming more frequent in older populations whose immunity has waned.

In general, the mild side effects of the MMR vaccine include pain and swelling at the injection site, cold-like symptoms, fever, swollen glands, headache, dizziness, rash, nausea, and vomiting. More moderate adverse effects are convulsions, arthritis, thrombocytopenia (bleeding disorder), Guillain-Barré, and rarely, severe allergic life-threatening reactions, deafness, comas, and permanent brain damage. The MMR vaccine has also been linked to autism.

Comments

As with the measles, Americans who were born before 1957 are considered immune to mumps because nearly everyone had it. It is normally a mild disease and complications are rare. This is not considered a high priority vaccine for many parents, due to its possible association of juvenile onset diabetes. People choosing this vaccine, though, should request it as a single shot rather than the three-in-one MMR.

Rubella (German Measles)
What Is Rubella?

German measles or rubella is a mild viral infection that used to be known as the *three-day measles*. Before the vaccine, rubella was common in children 5 to 9 years old. It occurs cyclically around the world every 6 to 9 years, most often in the late winter and spring. It is a contagious disease that is spread through close contact. There is an incubation period of 12 to 23 days.

Symptoms of Rubella

Symptoms of rubella begin with a low-grade fever, then swollen glands and fatigue for a few days. Rubella comes from the Latin for "little red," which describes a pink-colored rash that appears on the face and then spreads downward. It usually goes away on its own within 3 to 5 days. Occasionally a previously infected person can have the infection again; however, it usually provides lifelong immunity.

Complications of Rubella

Complications are rare, although up to three-quarters of women who contract rubella suffer from joint stiffness or arthritis that lasts for weeks, but may become chronic. Additional possible complications include diabetes, thrombocytopenic purpura (a blood condition that occurs in 1 out of 3,000 cases) and encephalitis (which occurs in 1 out of 6,000 cases). Because of the vaccine, infections are occurring in older age groups, among whom complications can be more serious.

The purpose of the vaccination is primarily to prevent Congenital Rubella Syndrome in babies. Congenital Rubella Syndrome occurs when a mother contracts rubella in her first trimester. If she is not immune to rubella (either through having the illness or through the vaccine), her fetus is at risk for birth defects. In addition, she may suffer a miscarriage. Twenty percent of babies exposed to this virus in utero are at risk for deafness, liver damage, and birth defects (especially in the eye, heart, or brain), including mental retardation. Currently, pregnant women are routinely given a blood test to confirm the presence of rubella antibodies which would protect them from infection.

How Common Is Rubella?

In the United States, there were over 57,000 reported cases of rubella in 1969. In 2002, there were 18 recorded cases. However, due to waning immunity, cases of rubella are rising among adolescents and adults, and can be more serious.

The last major rubella epidemic was in 1964–5, when there were 12.5 million rubella cases, including 20,000 babies born with congenital rubella syndrome.

Treatment of Rubella

Standard medicine has no treatment for rubella. The symptoms of fever do not respond to antibiotics or cough medicine, though supportive treatment, such as rest and fluids, are helpful. Homeopathy, naturopathy, traditional Chinese medicine, and chiropractics have all been useful in the treatment of rubella and in strengthening the body's natural ability to heal.

The Rubella Vaccine

Measles, mumps, and rubella (MMR) vaccines are given as a three-in-one shot of live viruses beginning at 1 year, with a second dose given at 4 to 6 years old. The vaccine is contraindicated in children who are allergic to eggs.

When administering the rubella vaccine on its own, most parents roughly follow the recommended schedule, giving it during baby's second year, with another dose around kindergarten.

Risks of the Vaccine

Side effects of the rubella vaccine by itself include arthritis, Guillain-Barré Syndrome, and thrombocytopenia, a low level of blood platelets, which help blood to clot.

During pregnancy, routine prenatal testing includes checking for rubella immunity. If a pregnant woman is found not to have proper immunity against rubella, she will be given a rubella shot after pregnancy, as the vaccination is contraindicated in pregnancy. I have treated several adult women patients who received their rubella vaccine immediately following childbirth. Several of these women began to suffer symptoms of arthritis following the shot. As always, if you decide to vaccinate, it is best to do it when you are feeling in full health to avoid any complications from the shot. Immediately after childbirth, most women are quite tired, so it is not an ideal time to receive a shot.

Mild side effects of the MMR vaccine include pain and swelling at the injection site, cold-like symptoms, fever, swollen glands, headache, dizziness, rash, nausea, and vomiting. More moderate adverse effects are convulsions, arthritis, thrombocytopenia (bleeding disorder), Guillain-Barré, and rarely, severe allergic life-threatening reactions, deafness, comas, and permanent brain damage. The MMR vaccine has also been linked to autism.

Comments

Rubella is a mild illness; however, there are complications that can occur during pregnancy, which makes this a vaccine to consider, especially for girls. For parents who will be vaccinating, I would give it before adulthood, because of its link to arthritis, which seems to be more common in adult women. With the MMR, I highly recommend the separated doses when vaccinating.

Chickenpox (Varicella)
What Is Chickenpox?

Chickenpox, also known as varicella, was a common childhood illness in the United States that affected as many as 4 million people a year before the vaccine. Nearly 90 percent of the population had chickenpox. Since the introduction of the vaccine, the number of cases has greatly diminished. Chickenpox is highly contagious and is related to shingles (herpes zoster), as both are part of the herpes family. Half of the cases of chickenpox occur in children from ages 5 to 9. It is considered a mild disease in childhood and a more severe one in adults. Usually, having the chickenpox gives one lifetime immunity. Chickenpox has an incubation period of 10 to 21 days.

Symptoms of Chickenpox

Symptoms of chickenpox include 1 to 2 days of mild general symptoms of fatigue, fever, and runny nose. This is followed by an intensely itchy rash that crusts over within 2 to 3 days. The rash appears in consecutive crops on the body, beginning on the head but occurring mainly on the torso and sometimes even in the mouth. It is usually extremely itchy and uncomfortable. Typically the illness lasts up to 2 to 3 weeks. More severe cases in adults can last up to several months.

Complications of Chickenpox

The most common complications include a bacterial skin infection in children, and pneumonia in adults. More severe problems include encephalitis (1 out of 4,000 to 10,000 cases), septicemia, and osteomyelitis. Less than 1 percent of children who get chickenpox suffer rare complications, though in both children and adults, severe complications are most likely to develop in those who have compromised immune systems due to other health problems. Before the introduction of the vaccine, there were approximately 100 deaths per year (more than half in adults).

The natural course following chickenpox infection is that the virus goes dormant in the nerve tract in the body. In an adult, the virus can become reactivated and appears as shingles, also in the herpes family. Shingles appears as painful and burning blisters, usually occurring on just one side of the body, and sometimes on the face and neck. The rash can last for 2 to 3 weeks, and a few people are left with a post-herpetic neuralgia, a debilitating pain. Shingles is more common in the elderly, and may be triggered by stress and a weakened immune system. Similar to chickenpox, an attack of shingles provides permanent immunity. In an article published in *International Journal of Toxicology*, Gary S. Goldman, Ph.D., wrote about the rates of shingles increasing since the chickenpox vaccine was mandated in 1995 but it is not clear if the two events are indeed related.

According to research from the British Public Health Laboratory Service, it is believed that when an adult is exposed to a child with chickenpox the adult's immune system receives a natural strengthening that offers antibody protection against shingles. In other words, being exposed to a child with chickenpox acts like a natural booster against shingles for the adult. The chickenpox vaccine and resultant fewer cases of the disease, it could result in increased cases of shingles in adults who would lose the natural protection.

Treatment of Chickenpox

Mainstream medicine uses calamine and caladryl lotion. Acyclovir, an antiviral medicine, is not used for healthy children but may be recommended for specific cases or high-risk groups who would be at risk for developing a severe infection.

An oatmeal bath can be very soothing. Homeopathic remedies may be used to provide relief for the itching and other symptoms.

The Chickenpox Vaccine

The chickenpox vaccine is made from live virus. The first dose is given at 12 to 15 months with a second dose at 4 to 6 years old. The vaccine is contraindicated in people who have allergy to gelatin or neomycin (antibiotic), or suffered a severe reaction to a previous chickenpox vaccine.

In addition to the rare complications from the disease, the CDC justifies the chickenpox vaccine because "children miss an average of 5 to 6 days of school when they have varicella and caregivers miss 3 to 4 days of work to care for their sick children." Widespread use of vaccine, however, may shift disease susceptibility to older populations, and the CDC is already noting the variable effectiveness of the vaccine—44 percent against the disease generally, and 86 percent against moderate or severe forms of the disease.

Risks of the Vaccine

Local reactions to the vaccine include pain, redness, and swelling (in 20 percent of cases), rash (in 4 percent or cases), and fever. The Vaccine Adverse Events Reporting System (VAERS) reports side effects including Guillain-Barré Syndrome, shingles, shock, encephalitis, blood disorders, and, in rare instances, death.

Comments

Because chickenpox is seen as a fairly harmless infection in most children, this is not a priority vaccine among many parents. Furthermore, the probable loss of protection against shingles in adults who are around children who have chickenpox could prove to have disastrous public health consequences in the years to come.

Hepatitis A

What Is Hepatitis A?

The hepatitis A virus (HAV) is well-known to travelers who have become infected after eating contaminated food. Because the virus is found in the stool of the infected person, this is known as the fecal-oral route. Hepatitis A can also be spread through diaper changes at daycare centers. For this reason, frequent handwashing is imperative after diaper changes, using the toilet, and before eating. If you or your child has come into contact with HAV, the U.S. Department of Health advises that an immune globulin shot that offers short-term protection be given within 2 weeks. The time of highest communicability is 2 weeks before the onset of symptoms. The incubation period is 28 days.

Symptoms of Hepatitis A

Hepatitis A usually lasts approximately 2 months and includes symptoms of fever, fatigue, loss of appetite, nausea, diarrhea, abdominal pain, dark urine, and jaundice. Up to 70 percent of children who contract hepatitis A have no symptoms and it usually goes undetected. Adults have symptoms more often than children. Once you have had hepatitis A, you maintain a lifelong immunity. Death is rare, with a mortality rate of 0.6 percent; most of these deaths occur in adults over age 49.

Complications of Hepatitis A

Up to 15 percent of people with hepatitis A can experience continued symptoms over a 6- to 9-month period. Otherwise, there is no long-term or chronic infection complication.

How Common Is Hepatitis A?

Hepatitis A is more common in other areas of the world, where close to 100 percent of people have antibodies to HAV. According to the CDC, approximately 30 percent of Americans are immune to HAV due to prior infection. Hepatitis A is more common in areas of poor hygiene and sanitation. Within the United States, most cases of HAV happen in the West and Southwest from local community outbreaks or from close personal contact within a household.

The Hepatitis A Vaccine

The vaccine was licensed for use in 1996. The hepatitis A vaccine is recommended to be given to children in two doses: the first dose given between 1 year and 18 months, with a second dose given 6 to 12 months after the first. The hepatitis A vaccine is also recommended for travelers in HAV-endemic areas and within 14 days after exposure. Protection may not be complete until 1 month following vaccination. It is given to children older than 1 year old with two doses given with a minimum interval between the first and booster doses of 6 months.

While many people support a mandatory hepatitis A vaccine for children, critics stress that HAV does not cause chronic infection, has a low mortality rate, especially among children, and is often asymptomatic in children. In addition, exposure to hepatitis A provides lifelong immunity compared to the vaccine, which provides a temporary protection. According to the National Vaccine Information Center, there have been no long-term reports studying the effects of the hepatitis A vaccine either given on its own or with other vaccines.

Risks of the Vaccine

Hepatitis A vaccines carry the risk of side effects, including headache, fatigue, joint pain, diarrhea, jaundice, vomiting and local reactions (50 percent) of tenderness, redness and swelling. More severe reactions such as Guillain-Barré Syndrome, anaphylactic shock, convulsions, multiple sclerosis, and death have also been reported.

Comments

Because hepatitis A is uncommon in the United States and usually is asymptomatic in children, I am not sure why this vaccine is recommended in the United States. The risks of the vaccine outweigh the benefits.

Meningococcal (Meningitis)
What Is Meningococcal Meningitis?

Meningitis is an inflammation of the covering of the brain or spinal cord (spinal meningitis) caused by either a virus or bacteria. The viral form is less severe, often requires no treatment, and is the most common form of meningitis in the United States. Bacterial meningitis is considered a serious health threat, and is caused by the *Neisseria meningitidis* (meningococcus), *Hemophilus influenza* type b (Hib), and *Streptococcus pneumoniae* (pneumococcus) strains. Hib is the most common infection in children under age 6 (see Hib vaccine). *Neisseria meningitidis* (meningococcus) is more common in children and adolescents 2 to 18 years old. It is not transmitted through casual contact nor is it as contagious as the flu, but is spread through close contact, such as kissing.

Symptoms of Meningococcal Meningitis

Symptoms of meningitis can progress rapidly within a few hours and include nausea, vomiting, headache, high fever, and stiff neck in children over age 2. In babies, symptoms of irritability, drowsiness and poor feeding are more characteristic.

Complications of Meningococcal Meningitis

Complications occur in 11 to 19 percent of cases and include hearing loss, convulsions, and brain damage. There are less than 2,600 cases a year of meningococcal meningitis, with a 10 percent death rate.

How Common Is Meningococcal Meningitis?

Meningococcal infection is more common in people with a weakened immune system, or no spleen, and those living in crowded living conditions, such as college students. However, the report from the CDC states that "college freshman, particularly those who live in dormitories, are at modestly increased risk relatives to other persons their age."

Treatment of Meningococcal Meningitis

Bacterial meningitis is treated with antibiotics and supportive therapy. Early intervention is important.

The Meningococcal Vaccine

There are three vaccines for bacterial meningitis: Hib (Haemophilus influenzae type B), pneumococcus, and meningococcus. The Hib and pneumococcal vaccines are routinely recommended for children; the meningococcal vaccine is not part of the childhood immunization schedule but is recommended for college students. The current meningococcal vaccine, MCV4 (Menactra), contains two of three of the most common strains of meningococcus the United States.

Risks of the Vaccine

The vaccine has its share of side effects, such as pain at the injection site, fever, and serious neurological disorders such as Guillain-Barré Syndrome. According to the CDC Recommendations of the Advisory Committee on Immunization Practices in 2000, "The risk for meningococcal disease among college students is low; therefore, vaccination of all college students, all freshmen, or only freshmen who live in dormitories or residence halls is not likely to be cost-effective for society as a whole."

Comments

Although bacterial meningitis is a serious illness, and the vaccine is recommended for college students by the CDC, there are not many overriding benefits to this vaccine considering the low rates of the disease in the designated population.

Human Papillomavirus (HPV)

What Is HPV?

One of the most recent vaccines to be added to the list is the Human Papillomavirus (HPV) vaccine, known as Gardasil. HPV, the most common sexually transmitted disease in the United States, has been linked to genital warts and cervical cancer.

Symptoms of HPV

Most often, people do not know they are infected because most cases of HPV have no symptoms. Eventually the virus goes away on its own. When symptoms do occur, they appear in the genital area, as single or clustered soft, sometimes cauliflower-shaped, wart-like growths.

Complications of HPV

There are more than 100 types of human papillomavirus, 30 of which are considered sexually transmitted diseases. Fifteen of these are linked to cervical cancer (in 70 percent of cases), anal cancer (in 30 to 50 percent of cases), and head and neck cancer (in 10 percent of cases). The risk for cervical cancer is increased with the use of the birth control pill for more than 5 years, chlamydia, herpes, HIV infection, and cigarette smoking.

How Common Is HPV?

HPV is a common infection that affects over 50 percent of sexually active men and women at some time in their lives.

Some women learn they have HPV from the results of an abnormal Pap test, a routine test performed in a gynecological exam, which can detect changes in the cervix. Following an abnormal Pap, a more sensitive test known as the HPV DNA can determine if these changes were caused by HPV. With repeat Pap smears, up to 90 percent of women will have normal tests within 1 to 2 years, without any recourse. Routine Pap screening, along with early intervention and treatment, can prevent the growth of HPV infection and reduce the rates of invasive cervical cancer. HPV infections can also be prevented or minimized by avoiding sexual contact or decreasing the number of sexual partners. Condoms provide some protection.

In general, deaths from cervical cancer, which account for less than 1 percent of all cancer deaths in the United States, have decreased by over 70 percent due to routine Pap smears. Precancerous cervical cells can take decades to develop into cancer. Everyone agrees that the HPV vaccine is not a substitute for routine Pap smears.

The HPV Vaccine (Gardasil)

The vaccine, Gardasil, contains the protein from only four types of HPV, two of them (HPV types 16 or 18) known to cause approximately 70 percent of cervical cancers. The other two types cause 90 percent of genital warts. The HPV vaccine does not protect against the other dozen cancer-causing HPV types.

The recent recommendations from the health department regarding the vaccine schedule note that the vaccine would be the most effective before sexual activity begins. For this reason, doctors give the vaccination to 11 to 12 year old girls, with "catch-up" vaccines given to females up through 26 years old. It is given in three doses within 1 year. The vaccine is not recommended for existing infections, but may be given to women 26 years or younger who have an abnormal Pap screen, positive HPV test, or genital warts.

Risks of the Vaccine

According to the Vaccine Adverse Event Reporting system, there have been hundreds of reports of vaccine reactions to Gardasil within months of its being licensed. Side effects of the vaccine include painful local reactions at the site of the vaccine, as well as moderate to severe neurological complaints that include numbness, tingling, twitching, fainting, seizures, vision and speech disorders, Guillain-Barré Syndrome, and collapse. Pain and neurological symptoms following the shot probably stem from the use of aluminum adjuvants in the vaccine. Aluminum is also used in other vaccines. This vaccine also contains polysorbate 80, which has been linked to infertility in mice. In addition, there have been reports of pregnant women who received the HPV vaccine; some experienced miscarriages and others had fetal abnormalities. Finally, a few women who received the vaccine have died.

Religious conservatives have been critical of the vaccine as it conflicts with the message of abstaining from sex. Other critics cite a lack of information on the vaccine. The vaccine's long-term effects on young girls, the duration of protection, and its effect on fertility are unknown. In addition, it is not known whether or not it may interact with other vaccines. National Vaccine Information Center health policy analyst Vicky Debold, R.N., Ph.D., recommended that girls should be vaccinated in a reclining position because of reports of fainting and collapse following the shot. In addition, it was preferable that patients not drive themselves home after receiving the shot.

Comments

The more I read about HPV, the less it seemed a menacing diagnosis when one considers that it is the most common sexually transmitted infection, often has no symptoms, and usually goes away without any recourse. In addition, remarkable strides have been made with early intervention of precancerous changes in the prevention of cervical cancer. All of these factors do not justify the need for another new vaccine that already is proving to have more risks than benefits.

Tuberculosis

What Is Tuberculosis?

Tuberculosis (TB) is a bacterial infection caused by *Mycobacterium tuberculosis*. Also known as consumption, phthisis, and white plague, it affected great numbers of children in the nineteenth century. As standards in living, sanitation, and medical care have improved, the disease has decreased in severity.

TB predominantly affects the lungs, though it can affect other parts of the body as well. It is contagious and transmitted by repeated or prolonged exposure to an infected person. An infected child can come down with the disease weeks or even years following exposure. An adult who has an active form of the disease was most likely infected years earlier.

Symptoms of Tuberculosis

There are different forms of tuberculosis. Primary pulmonary tuberculosis is the initial infection in a child. Usually, the child has no complaints and shows no signs of infection because the immune system is able to fight off and eradicate the infection. At that time, though, the child may have a positive tuberculin skin test. Most first infections resolve, and the child develops immunity. A positive PPD test (described below) can mean that your child may have been infected with TB, but it does not mean that your child has the disease. Only 10 percent of those infected go on to develop active tuberculosis.

Complications of Tuberculosis

In progressive tuberculosis, the symptoms resemble a process of "wasting away," and include weight loss, fever, loss of appetite, cough, and fatigue. Reactivation tuberculosis, yet another form of TB, follows the primary infection, sometimes years later, when inactive bacteria that have remained dormant in the lungs become active again. Following stress or a weakening of the immune system, the bacteria become activated and progressive. Reactivation TB can occur in both adolescents and adults, with symptoms that include fatigue, weight loss, loss of appetite, cough (occasionally with blood), fever, chills, and night sweats.

How Common Is Tuberculosis?

In the United States, TB is less prevalent than it used to be and is considered a curable disease. Around the world, though, TB infects more than a billion people, and in developing countries, TB is still the number one cause of death. By the 1920s, the rate of TB was declining in industrialized countries due to improvements in public health and standard of living; however, in the mid-1980s, the United States witnessed a resurgence of TB, due to higher rates of immune-deficiency illnesses, such as AIDS, infected immigrants, and the emergence of drug-resistant forms of TB. Despite this, early diagnosis and treatment have been successful in the treatment of tuberculosis.

Treatment of Tuberculosis

A child with a positive PPD test may have no symptoms, but will still be sent for a chest x-ray, which is usually normal. According to standard protocols, a positive PPD test, without any signs or symptoms of the disease, often warrants preventive treatment to kill germs that have the potential to become activated. The most common treatment is isoniazid (INH), which is given for 9 months. Those with active TB infection and symptoms are usually given a combination of drugs over 9 months. In earlier times, children and adults with tuberculosis were sent away to sanitariums to allow the body to rest and heal, and to avoid infecting others. In addition to standard treatments, homeopathy and other forms of alternative medicine can be helpful in the treatment of tuberculosis.

The Tuberculosis Skin Test (Mantoux Test)

The TB skin test, known as the Mantoux or PPD test, is the current main method for detecting tuberculosis. A small amount of tuberculin (purified, protein-derivative, or PPD) is injected in the skin on the forearm. Within 48 to 72 hours, the child must revisit a medical professional for examination of the forearm. The PPD test is read as positive when there is a reaction around the site of the injection. A second type of test, the tine test, uses multiple pins that contain tuberculin. However, the tests are not always reliable, as sometimes there are inaccurate readings. The pitfalls of the tests are the false positive and false negative results. For this reason, the tuberculin skin test is recommended only for high-risk children.

Children at high risk for TB are those who are exposed to an infected adult on a prolonged or repeated basis. In general, high-risk groups include people in prison, the homeless, alcoholics, IV drug abusers, those who are HIV-positive, and immigrants from countries with high rates of TB—some regions in Latin America (including Mexico), Asia, the Middle East, India, Vietnam, China, the Philippines, and Africa. To minimize exposure, avoid contact with people who have active infections.

A person can have a positive reaction despite not having tuberculosis; this is a false-positive skin test. False-positive tests can occur if the person has had another type of mycobacterial infection (non-tuberculous), a circumstance more common in HIV-positive people and those who have had a tuberculosis vaccine (BCG). On the other hand, the skin test can be false-negative in the elderly; in people with weak immune systems; in people who have cancer; in those who have had a recent viral infection such as influenza, measles or mumps; people with recent TB infection; in those who have had a recent measles, mumps, rubella vaccine (MMR); and people on steroids or immune-suppressive drugs. Side effects to the Mantoux test include itching, redness, peeling, and rash around the site of the injection. On rare occasions, people can have a generalized allergic reaction within 24 hours of the test, with hives and difficulty breathing. Also rarely, the site of the injection can have severe blisters, ulcers, and necrosis (death of the tissue).

Alternatives to the Standard TB Skin Test

Some families have refused the TB skin test on several grounds, based on the possible side effects as well as reports that the skin test is totally inaccurate and can lead to false-positive or false-negative results, and lack of confidence in the ability of medical professionals properly interpret a skin test.

As a substitute for the skin test, there are several alternatives to test for TB. According to recent guidelines published by the CDC, the Quanti-FERON TB Gold test (QFT-G) is a simple blood test that can be performed in all cases in which the TB skin test is indicated. This test has the advantage of requiring only one visit to the doctor's office, instead of the traditional 2-day follow-up with the skin test for a reading. However, the sensitivity of the test on children is still unknown. The QFT-G is similar to the skin test in that both can be used for screening but not diagnosis of severity of disease. If either test has a positive result, further evaluation is required.

In addition, a sputum AFB test for tuberculosis has been accepted by schools and in the workplace. The sputum test is performed by coughing up mucous from the lungs. The sample is sent the laboratory to rule out tuberculosis. The sputum test may not be entirely accurate either.

The Tuberculosis Vaccine

The tuberculosis vaccine is the BCG (Bacille Calmette-Guérin) and it is not given in the United States. There have been questions regarding its effectiveness. Side effects include local pain, swollen glands, discharging ulcer, abscesses, tuberculosis, and a number of deaths. Following the vaccine, a person will have a positive TB test for a while. A positive reaction on a skin test after someone has recently had the BCG vaccine is not considered reliable.

Comments

With the drawbacks of the Mantoux skin test, I am encouraged by alternative screening tests, especially the QuantiFERON TB Gold blood test, that are available for children who are at high risk for tuberculosis.

Anthrax

What Is Anthrax?

September 11, 2001, and the events immediately following placed biological and germ warfare, especially with anthrax and smallpox, at the forefront of national consciousness. Anthrax is an infectious disease caused by the bacterium *Bacillus anthracis*. It mostly occurs in wild and domestic animals such as cattle, sheep, goats, camels, and antelopes. There are three forms of the disease: cutaneous (skin), inhaled (lungs), and ingested (gastrointestinal). Humans can contract anthrax by coming in contact with infected animals via an open skin wound, by inhaling anthrax airborne spores, or by eating undercooked meat from infected animals. The inhalation form of the disease is most severe, and is usually fatal.

Symptoms of Anthrax

Anthrax symptoms vary depending on how the disease was contracted, but symptoms usually occur within 7 days. Skin infection begins as a raised itchy bump that resembles an insect bite, but within 1 to 2 days progresses into a painless ulcer, with a characteristic black area in the center. Nearby lymph glands may swell. With inhalation anthrax, an exposed individual develops flu-like symptoms (which can include fatigue, muscle and body aches, fever, and cough), which can last 2 to 3 days. Following these initial symptoms, the exposed person improves and begins to feel better. After several days, new symptoms appear, including severe breathing problems with bloody, frothy mucous, chest pain, sweating, and shock. The intestinal form of anthrax includes symptoms of nausea, loss of appetite, vomiting, and fever. Subsequently abdominal pain, vomiting of blood, and severe diarrhea occur.

The Anthrax Vaccine

An anthrax vaccine has been licensed for use in humans, and is reported to be 93 percent effective in protecting against anthrax. The Department of Defense has begun mandatory vaccination of all active-duty military personnel who might be involved in a conflict.

Risks of the Vaccine

The anthrax vaccine is considered experimental, and American troops were forced to take it beginning in 1998. According to the Military Vaccine Education Center, an organization that aids soldiers who have been injured by vaccines, symptoms from the anthrax vaccination include severe fatigue, weakness, migraines, tremors, tumors, seizures, heart conditions, and death.

Comments

The benefits of this vaccine do not outweigh the risks.

Smallpox

What Is Smallpox?

Smallpox was once believed to be completely eradicated, but outbreaks are still a possible, though rare, occurrence. A viral disease unique to humans, smallpox can only be propagated through person-to-person contact. The infection is spread by the inhalation of air droplets or aerosols. The disease can lead to death.

Symptoms of Smallpox

The incubation period from time of exposure until symptoms develop is 12 to 14 days. After the incubation period, the person experiences a fever, severe aching, and weakness. Severe abdominal pain and delirium are also possible. Two to 3 days later, a papular rash (pimples) develops over the face, then spreads to the extremities, turning into a vesicular rash (clear fluid-filled blisters), and finally to a pustular rash (yellowish pus-filled blisters) deeply imbedded in the skin. Eventually scabs form leaving deep, pitting scars. Chickenpox is very similar-looking and can be mistaken in the first 2 to 3 days of the rash. However, chickenpox lesions generally develop in crops over several days and are much more superficial.

The Smallpox Vaccine

The CDC recommends routine vaccinations only for laboratory staff who may be exposed to the virus. The vaccination poses risks and complications, and the overall stock is low, as the facilities that made it were dismantled after 1980 when smallpox was considered eradicated.

Risks of the Vaccine

The smallpox (vaccinia) vaccine is a live virus that has a high rate of side effects. For months following the vaccine, children may suffer with fever, irritability, rash, lack of energy, and swollen glands. The site of the vaccine is contagious with live virus and a person who is recently vaccinated can transmit the virus to other areas of the body, which causes lesions to form. Severe side effects are likely and include neurological reactions such as encephalitis.

Comments

There is no benefit to this vaccine at this time.

Travel Vaccines

In past centuries, there have been epidemics of cholera, typhoid, and yellow fever, and other similar infectious diseases in our country. Along with many childhood illnesses, there has been a decline in the frequency and severity of these diseases due to improved hygiene, sanitation, and nutrition, as well as the availability of vaccinations and more effective treatments. However, these diseases are still prevalent in many other countries, especially in Africa, South America, and Asia. When traveling to these countries, additional vaccines may be recommended.

The yellow fever vaccine is required for travel to sub-Saharan Africa and tropical South America and the meningococcal vaccine is required for travel to Saudi Arabia, especially during the Hajj, or pilgrimage, when there will be many people in close quarters. The CDC also maintains a list of recommended vaccinations and preventive medications, designated for travelers and listed by country. It includes such factors as time spent in rural areas, season, standard of health, and prior immunizations.

In addition to getting the recommended vaccinations, follow these general guidelines whenever traveling to prevent exposure to contaminated food and water:

- Drink bottled water when possible. Carbonated is safer than flat water.
- Otherwise, drink water that has vigorously boiled for at least 1 minute.
- Avoid ice, unless you are certain it is made from clean water.

- Eat cooked food, preferably still hot. Do not eat raw vegetables (including salad) and fruit unless you peel them yourself. Avoid eating from street vendors.

Some of the vaccines that may be recommended for travel include:

Cholera

Cholera is an acute diarrheal illness caused by the bacterium *Vibrio cholerae*. Rare in the United States and other Western countries over the past century, cholera is more common in sub-Saharan Africa and the Indian subcontinent, where it predominantly affects young children. Breastfed infants are less affected. Cholera occurs usually in epidemics and is spread by contaminated water or food. The incubation period is 1 to 5 days. Drinking safe bottled water, eating cooked foods, and avoiding ice and eating from street vendors can decrease the incidence of contracting cholera.

SYMPTOMS: More often it is a mild illness (sometimes without symptoms). Only 5 percent of cases are severe, with the characteristic symptoms of copious watery diarrhea, vomiting, and cramps. It can rapidly cause dehydration from loss of fluids, especially in children. Extreme cases result in death.

TREATMENT: Treatment consists of replacement of fluids and salt lost through diarrhea. Less important are antibiotics, which may decrease symptoms and shorten the course of the illness.

VACCINE: Currently there is no cholera vaccine available in the United States. There is an oral vaccine available in a few countries that provides temporary protection.

Malaria

Malaria is a common infectious disease caused by four types of malaria parasites. It is transmitted by the bite of the female *Anopheles* mosquito. It is widespread in developing countries located in the tropical and sub-tropical parts of the world, including Central and South America, Africa, the Indian subcontinent, Southeast Asia, and the Middle East. The incubation period following an infected mosquito bite is 10 days to 4 weeks.

SYMPTOMS: Symptoms of malaria include high fever, shaking chills, flu-like symptoms, headache, and vomiting. Complications include jaundice, and severe anemia, which can progress to complications in the brain and other organs. Some people suffer with malarial attacks of intermittent fevers that can occur after months or years. There are 300 million acute cases a year and one million deaths, mostly in African children living south of the Sahara.

VACCINE: Instead of a vaccine, travelers in endemic areas use oral standard antimalarial medication, which is begun prior to travel. There are several types of medications that can be used. One of these, Lariam (Mefloquine), has side effects including nausea, vomiting, abdominal pain, dizziness, poor balance, insomnia, anxiety, depression, hallucinations and more. These occur in 15 percent of women and 8 percent of men. Children may require special dosage preparations based on weight, age and choice of medication. Additional precautions such as using insect repellant, use of mosquito bed nets, and wearing protective clothing are advised.

Typhoid Fever

Typhoid fever is a bacterial infection caused by Salmonella typhi. The bacteria reside in the bloodstream and intestines (feces) of infected people. Some people are carriers without symptoms. Typhoid fever is spread by exposure to food and water contaminated by an infected person or from raw sewage. It is found in Central and South America, Africa, Southeast Asia, and the Indian subcontinent. Because this illness is spread by person-to-person contact, one should use the same general precautions of hygiene and food handling as with cholera and hepatitis A. Well-known in the United States, Typhoid Mary was a healthy carrier who worked as a cook and was responsible for several typhoid outbreaks in the early 1900s.

SYMPTOMS: Symptoms of typhoid fever are sudden onset of continuous high fever, weakness, headache, loss of appetite, diarrhea (also constipation) and sometimes a rash of flat, rose-colored spots. Complications include intestinal hemorrhage or perforation, encephalitis, and dehydration.

Typhoid fever commonly affects children from 5 to 19 years old. In 2000, typhoid fever affected over 17 million people worldwide with 600,000 deaths. When treated with antibiotics, the mortality rate decreases to 1 percent.

VACCINE: There are two vaccines available for typhoid fever. Vivotif is an oral vaccine that contains a live weakened strain of the bacteria. It is not given to children less than 6 years old. Typhim Vi is a single-dose injectable vaccine that is licensed for children 2 years and older. For children less than 2 years old, it is imperative to use extra precautions with hygiene and food handling. Because there is no option for vaccination for families with infants, many people are interested in using homeopathic and other forms of natural prevention against typhoid fever.

RISKS OF VACCINE: The oral vaccine Vivotif has side effects of abdominal bloating or queasy feeling as well as vomiting, cramps, diarrhea, skin rash, fever, or headache. It may interact with other vaccines and medications. Side effects of the injectable vaccine, Typhim Vi, include pain and swelling at the site of the injection, fever, and headache. The vaccines are not considered totally effective.

Yellow Fever

Yellow fever is a viral illness that is spread from the bite of an infected mosquito. The disease infects both humans and monkeys. Often striking in epidemic proportions, yellow fever is more common in Africa and South America. It is considered a required vaccination for travel in some regions, although it rarely occurs in travelers. It has an incubation period of 3 to 6 days.

SYMPTOMS: Yellow fever has several distinct disease phases. The initial acute period consists of nausea, vomiting, fever (with slow pulse), shivers, muscle ache (back), headache, loss of appetite, and sometimes jaundice. The name "yellow" fever comes from the jaundice symptoms. Although most people improve and the condition resolves after 4 days, 15 percent experience a more severe phase with vomiting, abdominal pain, bleeding, and kidney failure. Half of these patients do not survive. Treatment consists of oral rehydration fluids and supportive measures. There are about 200,000 cases a year with 30,000 deaths, according to the World Health Organization.

VACCINE: The yellow fever vaccine is considered 95 percent effective. It is not advised for people with allergies to eggs, chicken or gelatin, people with HIV, and people on certain medications such as steroids or chemotherapy.

RISKS OF VACCINE: Side effects of the vaccine include fever, pain at the site of injection, flu-like symptoms, rash, allergies, behavior changes, and convulsions. Mild side effects occur in approximately 25 percent of cases and include headaches, muscle aches, and low fever. On rare occasions there have been instances of multiple organ system failure, encephalitis, and death. The vaccine is not recommended in infants younger than 9 months old. As with other illnesses that are spread by mosquitoes, it is important to use precautions that prevent mosquito bites. A waiver letter prior to travel can be obtained for those in whom the vaccine is contraindicated. This includes infants less than 9 months old, pregnant women, and those with egg allergy, HIV infection, or weakened immune system.

CHAPTER 6

Alternatives to the Standard

Vaccine Schedule

Many parents have told me that once baby is born and the doctor visits begin, it seems that everything becomes routine, including the vaccination schedule. Furthermore, most believe that vaccinations are mandatory for entry into school. With more information available and questions raised on the safety of vaccines, however, more parents are realizing they have choices available to them and that not every vaccine is necessary for entry into school. As a result, pediatricians and other healthcare practitioners are increasingly confronted with patients who want to diverge from the standard vaccine protocol, preferring to vaccinate slowly, selectively, or not at all. I receive many calls from families nationally who are in search of practitioners who are willing to work with families who have chosen not to vaccinate, or prefer a selective shot schedule, or who desire a frank discussion to help decide what to do. There are various organizations that offer information about like-minded practitioners, such as the National Center for Homeopathy (http://nationalcenterforhomeopathy.org) and the Holistic Pediatric Assocation (http://www.hpakids.org).

No Vaccinations

Most families I've met who decided not to vaccinate their children at all have spent time researching the various points of view and have seriously considered the risks and benefits of not vaccinating their child. The most common reason I hear from parents who have chosen not to vaccinate is they are concerned about adverse effects from the vaccinations.

If more children are not being vaccinated, this lowers the herd immunity in the community, which will make all children more susceptible to getting these diseases. In countries like Sweden, West Germany, England, and Japan, where the pertussis vaccination rates fell to 30 percent in the 1970s, it caused the population to lose herd immunity within 3 years. As a result, whooping cough rates increased. In the case of pertussis, the herd immunity threshold is 92 to 94 percent; that is, 92 to 94 percent of the population needs to be vaccinated in order for the vaccine to also protect unvaccinated people.

It would be naïve to take the "it won't happen to us" attitude. It is possible for any child, even a vaccinated one, to succumb to a serious infectious illness. If you are considering not vaccinating your child, it is important to familiarize yourself ahead of time with the risk your child has of getting each illness, the symptoms of each illness, and the options for treatment. For natural immune strengthening tips, see page 116.

Selective Shot Schedules

For parents who are interested in a slower or selective vaccination schedule for their children, there are various options available for delaying or reducing the number of shots. A common concern among families on separated vaccines is the insurance reimbursement vesus out-of-pocket expenses. In my office, we offer separated thimerosal-free shots and accept most insurance plans. Most insurance companies have an immunization fee schedule that covers both separated and combined vaccines. However, providers vary so it is best to speak to your practitioner's office and your insurance agent for further information regarding the details of your plan.

START AT A LATER AGE: Many parents are choosing to begin the shots when their baby is older, often at 6 months or 1 year, when the baby's immune system is stronger. According to vaccine expert Dr. Viera Scheibner, in the early 1970s, there were 37 infant deaths after the DTP vaccine was introduced. As a result, from 1975 to 1980, Japan delayed giving children the older DTP immunization until 2 years old, which resulted in a significant decrease in vaccine side effects, including sudden infant death syndrome (SIDS) which fell to three deaths. Also, the mortality rate from whooping cough in babies had dropped significantly, which is ironic because the vaccine is supposed to prevent whooping cough (pertussis). In overall infant mortality, Japan moved from 17th to 1st place in the world in the mid-1970s. By 1988, the Japanese began to vaccinate at 3 months old and the rate of SIDS in babies less than 1 year old rose to 0.33 percent in 1992, which was a sharp incline compared to 0.07 percent in 1980. The DTP is no longer being used as it has been associated with severe vaccine injuries and death. It has been replaced by the newer DTaP.

CHOICE OF VACCINATIONS: Become informed. Evaluate your child's risk or susceptibility (for instance, daycare setting versus staying at home). This can help you decide which vaccines are a priority. For example, some parents feel strongly against giving the hepatitis B vaccine to their infant if there are no risk factors in either parent for hepatitis B. They may choose to postpone the vaccine until the teen years. From my own experience, when families who are "on the fence" meet with their pediatricians, the most common vaccinations that pediatricians encourage for the first year are usually Hib meningitis and pertussis (part of the DTaP).

MAKE YOUR OWN SCHEDULE: Once you decide which vaccinations are right for your child, discuss with your practitioner a timeframe for how to proceed. Many parents aim to give one shot at a time (not possible in the DTaP). Allow time in between the shots and stagger them accordingly. This avoids overloading the body at one time. Waiting also allows the body to recover in between the shots, and may minimize a possible vaccine reaction. You may have to search for a little while to find a practitioner who offers the shots separately; however, by your requests, you can create a demand for separate shots.

Exemptions from the Standard Schedule

When my sons began kindergarten, I received their registration packets complete with medical forms and a vaccination history to fill out. When a child is school age (even for preschool), you will be asked about your child's medical history, including dates of vaccinations. Many parents are surprised to find out that although vaccinations are seemingly compulsory, exemptions and waivers do exist.

If you have opted to either vaccinate selectively or not at all, you will need to be able to explain your choice. In the United States, the immunization laws differ in each state. It is important to be familiar with your state's immunization law, legal vaccine requirements, and recommended vaccines. For example, some states may not require the mumps vaccine, although it is recommended along with the required measles and rubella shots (MMR). If you or your child has already had an illness such as chickenpox, you can probably be exempted from the vaccination if you are able to show proof of immunity from a blood test.

Some families who have opted for an exemption have encountered resistance when presenting a waiver. However, usually after a brief explanation of the vaccine law in each particular state, most school administrators are willing to work with the family and most parents report they simply signed a waiver provided by the school. Often opposition is encountered because the school nurse or administrator may not even be aware that exemptions exist. Each state has different requirements with specific guidelines for exemptions. The following types are available to parents in most states:

PERSONAL, PHILOSOPHICAL OR CONSCIENTIOUSLY HELD BELIEFS: In some states you must waive all vaccinations in order to be allowed to use this exemption; in other states, selective vaccination is acceptable.

MEDICAL: All states permit medical exemptions. The patient's doctor must write why the child is medically unable to receive a vaccination, and that receiving a shot would be harmful. In some states, the state health department intervenes to evaluate the case.

PROOF OF IMMUNITY: If your child has had the illness or been previously vaccinated, and can demonstrate proof of immunity from the levels of antibodies in a blood test, some states will permit an exemption.

RELIGIOUS: Most states allow one to file an exemption based on beliefs that compulsory vaccinations would violate their religious rights. An example would be the Christian Scientists who trust in God's power of healing, and consider medical intervention unnecessary. Families usually are obliged to offer proof of affiliation with their organization.

Homeopathic Alternatives to Vaccines (Nosodes)

Long before vaccines, blood tests, and x-rays, practitioners sought ways to ward off diseases and human sufferings. Amber was used for generations in European countries to soothe teething infants. Angelica root was used to ward off the plague. By the late 1700s, medicine had begun to change. Dr. Edward Jenner had begun experimenting successfully with a vaccination against smallpox. Dr. Samuel Hahnemann, the father of homeopathy, made tremendous strides with homeopathic medicine as a prophylaxis during a scarlet fever outbreak. One of the first books on the results of vaccination was published in 1897 by J. Compton Burnett, M.D., a physician and homeopath. In his book *Vaccinosis* he wrote about the treatment for adverse effects and chronic disease as a result of the smallpox vaccination.

Homeopathic medicine is based on the principle that minute doses of a substance can heal the very symptoms it would cause if taken in its natural undiluted state. The principle, known as the "law of similars" or like cures like, states that a substance can cause symptoms in large amounts, yet have healing properties in microdoses. For instance, a common homeopathic medicine, *Allium cepa*, made from red onion, is used to treat watery runny nose and red eyes that come from a cold or hay fever—the very symptoms red onion would cause if you were cutting it in the kitchen. Homeopathic medicine is a form of natural holistic medicine that can be used to treat conditions in both children and adults. It is safe, nontoxic, and without side effects.

Due to its great success in the prevention and treatment of epidemics, homeopathic medicine become widespread in the 1800s. American medical doctors started to use homeopathy in their practices during the cholera epidemic of 1849. By 1900, there were over a hundred homeopathic hospitals in the U.S. alone. The American Medical Association (AMA) began in direct response to the popularity and success of homeopathic medicine, and effectively forced this once very mainstream medical practice to the sidelines of U.S. healthcare, albeit temporarily. Today homeopathy is used worldwide and is once again becoming popular in the United States. Interestingly, the only time homeopathy and conventional medicine (allopathy) "appear" to be similar is along the subject of vaccines—in which both employ small doses of a substance to prevent a later infection by that substance.

Different from standard vaccinations, homeopathic prophylaxis, as it is known, has originally been documented to offer immunity if given during an epidemic, for short-term protection. The medicine would need to be repeated in the event of other exposures in the future. As experience grew with more data compiled over the years, the idea of homeopathic prophylaxis as a long term protection has been used by some homeopaths. In keeping with the common adage "Less is more," many practitioners prefer to still treat only when the need arises rather than routinely, as is done with the standard vaccination schedule.

In her book *Homeopathy in Epidemic Diseases* (published in 1967), Dorothy Shepherd, M.D., writes, "Believe me, it has been shown again and again that our medicines given intelligently and according to our law that "like cures like" do not only cure infectious diseases speedily and easily without the development of any complications, but they also prevent these same diseases. This is of great importance, particularly in the case of infants who have not enough stamina to stand up to an onslaught of whooping cough or measles or diphtheria, or infantile paralysis...." According to Dr. Shepherd, the homeopathic nosode *Pertussin* was given daily for 14 days to 364 children who had been exposed to whooping cough. None of the children developed it. In a polio outbreak, 82 people were given the homeopathic remedy *Lathyrus sativa*; again, there were no cases of illness.

In Hahnemann's time, when epidemics such as scarlet fever, cholera, and diphtheria were commonplace, homeopaths had ample evidence that their medicines provided significant protection from getting the illnesses. In his early research with homeopathy, Hahnemann verified that he was able to use the remedies to prevent and treat illness during outbreaks. He called his concept of finding the right remedy for an epidemic the Genus Epidemicus. He collected data on the signs and symptoms from several affected patients, and, by looking at the similar complaints in the patients, he was able to ascertain and decide on the appropriate choice of homeopathic medicine for that particular epidemic, which he would be able to prescribe en masse for prevention and treatment. Homeopaths would later realize that it was best to find the Genus Epidemicus for each epidemic, as the symptoms subtly change even if it is the same disease. Nowadays, it is not uncommon to hear homeopaths discussing the Genus Epidemicus for particular flu seasons.

According to the eminent American homeopath Carol Dunham, M.D. (1828–1877), "The selection of the prophylactic remedy must to some extent be governed by the nature of the epidemic, and therefore the best preventive cannot always be determined until the epidemic has appeared and its peculiar nature has been determined." In an attempt to appeal to the mainstream approach to vaccination, some homeopaths have expanded to a broad-spectrum homeopathic prophylaxis approach.

Called homeopathic *nosodes*, these medicines are prepared from specific diseases. Based on the theory of nosodes, in 1833, Dr. Constantine Hering suggested the use of the homeopathic remedy *Lyssinum* (made from the saliva of a rabid dog) in the treatment of rabies, decades before Pasteur was acknowledged for the rabies vaccine.

With time, homeopaths expanded the concept of a broad-spectrum use of homeopathic prophylaxis, employing nosodes that paralleled the conventional approach. To date a list of homeopathic medicines is employed by homeopathic practitioners to prevent or treat specific illnesses. Among the practitioner, the protocols vary—some prescribe in a vaccine schedule similar to the standards, while others prefer to treat at the time of an outbreak, as well as preventively for travel.

Homeopathic Nosodes for Travel

I subscribe to the classical homeopathic approach of using a homeopathic medicine as a prophylaxis when it is needed: for example, during an epidemic or for travel. My willingness to prescribe homeopathy prophylaxis for travel is based on excellent results that have been recorded by homeopathic practitioners for the past several centuries.

As a physician, I also provide standard medications and vaccines for diseases such as yellow fever, malaria, hepatitis A, and typhoid to patients before travel. In addition, many of my patients come to my office in search of homeopathic and natural alternatives to use during their travels. Although in mainstream medicine there aren't many current studies or data suggesting that homeopathic microdoses of hepatitis A, typhoid, malaria, yellow fever, salmonella typhi, and others can prevent these conditions, many of my patients still prefer to take homeopathic medicines on their travels in lieu of not doing anything or in conjunction with standard recommended procedures. Most report excellent success on their voyages.

I always caution everyone that no modality—whether a standard vaccine or homeopathic nosode—is ever 100 percent foolproof. For more information on alternative remedies and treatments you can use during your travels, see the Resource section in the back of this book to find a practitioner in your area.

CHAPTER 7

The Safe Shot Strategy

From the Hippocratic oath of "First do no harm" to the homeopathic aphorism, "The physician's highest and only calling is to make the sick healthy, to cure, as it is called," every practitioner's mission is to provide quality care to patients, and do no harm. The idea that vaccination, which is hailed as one of the greatest successes in public health, could be dangerous is an outrageous notion to most physicians. With more people recognizing that there can be side effects following a shot, parents are interested in taking measures to minimize if not prevent any health problems.

If you decide to vaccinate, make sure your child is in good health. If your child is sick or has been recently (in the past 2 weeks), I encourage the "wait until better" approach. If your child is cranky, fussy or not herself or himself, this may mean that the child could be getting sick: wait until he or she is better. If your child has been on antibiotics, wait at least 6 weeks until getting a shot. Antibiotics weaken the immune system, and it is not uncommon that children become sick soon after. Wait until your child is better.

For children who have chronic condition such as allergies, eczema, or recurrent ear infections, the timing of vaccination becomes more complex. Unfortunately, so many children live with chronic problems now that we also need to consider the possibility that the condition has been caused by or is connected to previous shots. I believe it is best to treat these underlying conditions, preferably with natural holistic medicine, before vaccinating again. Many parents bring their children to see me for a homeopathic medicine to help strengthen their child's constitution before getting a shot, with hopes that this will decrease the chance that the vaccine could aggravate the preexisting condition.

If you vaccinate your child, I would recommend using a safe shot strategy to prevent or at least minimize any possible adverse effects following a shot. The safe shot strategy is outlined in four steps.

1. Be familiar with the disease. Answer the following questions:
   a. What is the disease?
   b. Are there any complications?
   c. How is it treated?
   d. How common is it in the area where I live? In my country?
   e. What is the risk of my child contracting the disease?
2. Be informed about the vaccine
   a. What are the benefits of the shot?
   b. What are the risks?
3. What is the standard vaccine schedule?
   a. Know which shots will be coming up at your next doctor visit.
4. Is this the right time to give the shot?
   a. If your child is ill, delay the shot until he or she is better.
   b. If your child has chronic conditions that might affect the immune response, talk to your practitioner before the vaccination.
   c. If you child has recently taken antibiotics, steroids or other strong medications that weaken the immune system, wait several weeks until stabilized.
   d. Check your child's health before and after the shot. Contact your physician if your child shows signs of agitation, discomfort, or serious illness.

Based on this information, there are eight questions prepared by the National Vaccine Information Center. Before any vaccination, it is recommended that you answer the following eight questions compiled by the National Vaccine Information Center:

1. Is my child sick right now?
2. Has my child had a bad reaction to a vaccination before?
3. Does my child have a personal or family history of:
   - vaccine reactions
   - convulsions or neurological disorders
   - severe allergies
   - immune system disorders
4. Do I know if my child is at high risk of reacting?
5. Do I have full information on the vaccine's side effects?
6. Do I know how to identify a vaccine reaction?
7. Do I know how to report a vaccine reaction?
8. Do I know the vaccine manufacturer's name and lot number?

Recognizing Vaccine Reactions (Immediate and Delayed)

Patients often complain that a visit to the doctor feels rushed, with more emphasis on the technology such as lab tests, x-rays, and ultrasound than on the patient.

Since becoming a holistic physician, I spend more time with patients and take a more comprehensive patient history, which includes getting to know their likes and dislikes, health habits, and other relevant details about their lifestyles and personalities. As a result, I find I have become more cognizant of the subtleties and various ways children respond to medications. This includes any reactions from vaccinations.

Because homeopathy has so many remedies that can be prescribed for treatment beyond what conventional medicine can offer, I am less tolerant of the pain and discomfort shots can cause infants and children. For instance,

I received a phone call from Marina, a distraught mother who complained that her 9-month-old son, David, had been crying constantly for 7 days and nights since he received his round of shots. Her pediatrician had gently re-assured her that the discomfort would pass and told her to give him ibupro-fen in the interim. I saw them in my office, where I gave David homeopathic *Chamomilla* 200C for extreme fussiness and irritability. By the next day, he had stopped fussing, and both mother and baby were able to resume their usual daily activities.

I often have to remind parents that they know their children better than any practitioner. Observe your child. Especially with younger children, I usu-ally receive more information from observation and their cues rather than from direct questions, which are often leading and bias the answer. Questions such as, "Does your ear hurt?" already assume there is ear pain. Observe your child's signals and if he or she is not feeling well the day of the shots, post-pone them until the child feels better.

Sometimes there can be reactions following a vaccination. Those that happen immediately after a shot can include:
- Allergic Reactions (hives, shock)
- Shock, collapse
- High-pitched screaming (persistent crying)
- High temperature
- Excessive sleepiness
- Convulsions
- Redness, pain and swelling at the site of the shot

The more common reactions that I see in my patients are fussiness, fever, sleepiness, and local pain and swelling at the injection site. Many other vac-cine-related symptoms may occur days, weeks, or even months later, and go unnoticed and underreported. The longer the time between a reaction and a shot, the more unlikely you or your doctor will make the association. A week after getting the MMR shot, 5 year old Christian came down with cold symptoms and woke up the next day with swollen joints and severe bruising. His mother carried him into my office after he was diagnosed with a bleeding disorder, ITP (idiopathic thrombocytopenic purpura), and arthritis. Based on his history and symptoms, I prescribed *Rhus toxicodendron* and several other homeopathic medicines over a 1-month period, after which Christian healed without recourse to allopathic medications.

Although the specific risks of the vaccines are outlined in Chapter 5, delayed side effects that could occur include:

- Blood conditions (hemorrhaging, idiopathic thrombocytopenic purpura)
- Encephalitis (inflammation of the brain)
- Attention Deficit Hyperactivity Disorder
- Learning disorders
- Developmental delays
- Multiple sclerosis
- Arthritis
- Neurological conditions
- Guillain-Barré Syndrome (GBS), an autoimmune disease that attacks healthy tissue. It presents with progressive muscle weakness and can cause paralysis of the legs, arms, breathing muscles, and face. The paralysis can be temporary. GBS can occur following infections, surgery, and immunizations.
- Convulsions
- Diabetes mellitus
- Spastic colon
- Pharyngitis
- Otitis media (ear infections)
- SIDS
- Upper respiratory tract infection

Natural Treatment to Strengthen the Immune System

Because it is important that your child be healthy at the time of the shots, I prefer extra strengthening for the immune system before and immediately following the shot. Most pediatricians will recommend that you give your child such medications as acetaminophen, to reduce any fever or body ache. In general, many parents in my office practice prefer not to begin with standard medications as they can mask or suppress symptoms, which can make it difficult to determine if there is any reaction, and, if so, would make it harder to find a proper homeopathic medicine.

I recommend administering the following suggested list of remedies 7 days before and after the shot for general strengthening of the body. These may also reduce possible side effects following the vaccine. Of course, these remedies can be used at any time, whether or not you choose to vaccinate. At our office, we offer separated, thimerosal-free shots, and provide parents with information on the following regime. They can be used in mixed variations:

- Black Currant (a gemmotherapy herbal preparation for general strengthening) can be given on alternate days with Briar Rose
- Briar Rose (a gemmotherapy herbal preparation for children's ailments and immune strengthening)

and/or

- Vitamin C (less than 2 years of age: 100 mg once daily—over 2 years old, 250 mg once a day)
- Juice Plus or other whole-food nutritional products or natural child's vitamin

and/or

- Natural general immune strengthener for children

In our office, we prescribe the following homeopathic medicines on the day of the shot:

- *Ledum palustre* 30C—for puncture wounds; 3 pellets 1 hour before shot, and 2 doses after the shot (every 12 hours)

- *Arnica montana* 30C—for local swelling and soreness; 3 pellets given twice a day for 2 days following the shot
- *Thuja occidentalis* 30C—a general medicine for vaccine effects; 3 pellets twice a day for 3 days following the shot
- *Chamomilla* 30C—for fussiness following the shot; 3 pellets as needed
- Constitutional remedies—Homeopathy and other forms of holistic medicine can offer a remedy that is chosen specifically for your child to help strengthen or maintain health when needed. Consider seeing a practitioner in your area.

Administering Homeopathic Remedies

Homeopathic remedies come as round, chewable pellets or as quick-dissolve tablets, depending on the brand you purchase. Both types are sweet and pleasant tasting, which make them easy to administer to children. When possible, avoid touching the tablets with your fingers. Use a spoon.

ADULTS AND CHILDREN: The dosages described above are for use following the shots. For treatment of illness, take three pellets three times a day or as directed by your practitioner. In acute cases, take every hour until relieved. If you see no improvement after three doses, discontinue the remedy.

Adults and older children are encouraged to let the tablets dissolve under the tongue. Younger children can let them dissolve in their mouths. If your child is too small to take the remedy, place three pellets in a half a glass of water and let stand for 5 minutes. Although the hard pellets will not dissolve immediately, the water becomes medicated. Stir 10 times, and give 1 teaspoonful (or dropperful).

EATING AND DRINKING. Avoid eating or drinking 10 minutes (if possible) before and after taking your homeopathic remedy. With a baby or small child this is not always possible. Not to worry!

SUBSTANCES TO AVOID. During the time period that you are taking a remedy, it is best to avoid coffee, chocolate, camphor, eucalyptus, mint, and other strong-smelling substances (mint toothpaste is okay).

PERSISTENT OR WORSENING SYMPTOMS. If symptoms of illness persist more than 3 days or worsen, discontinue the remedy and consult your doctor.

IMPROVING SYMPTOMS. As your condition improves, take your homeopathic medicine less often (1 or 2 times a day). When you are substantially better, discontinue the medicine.

STORING AND TRAVELING. Store your homeopathic medicines away from electrical appliances, strong-smelling substances, and extremes of temperature.

For more information on treatment of symptoms such as fever and diarrhea, or specific conditions such as flu, chickenpox, measles, mumps, whooping cough, etc, see *Natural Baby and Childcare.*

Administering Gemmotherapy

Gemmotherapy herbal remedies are diluted herbs (1:10 strength) in a base of alcohol with glycerin and water. They are prepared in an amber glass bottle with a dropper. If your child is sensitive to alcohol, place the open bottle in 1 inch of slow boiling water for 5 minutes. Cool the bottle before screwing on the stopper. The shelf life without alcohol is approximately 3 weeks.

Gemmotherapy remedies are easy to administer. They can be given directly under the tongue, though most children prefer them in a beverage, such as water. Ideally, they should be taken one at a time in water. However, they can be taken together mixed in water or juice.

The dosage for infants is 5 to 8 drops. Give children ages 3 to 8 years old 12 to 15 drops, and older children and adults, 25 drops. The remedies can be used as often as 2 or 3 times per day during acute illness. Gemmotherapy is considered a professional line and is available through healthcare providers and selected pharmacies. Gemmos can be used in conjunction with each other (up to three at a time), with homeopathic medicines, and any other medicines. As with any remedy, use when needed, then discontinue.

Safe Shot Strategy for Travel Vaccinations

In addition to the standard vaccination schedule for children, various shots are recommended for travel in exotic places. For children or adults who are choosing to vaccinate before travel, it is important to consider using the same safe shot strategy that I recommend for general vaccines in childhood. I have patients who have experienced deleterious effects, some of them chronic, after receiving multiple vaccines for travel at the same time.

What's Right for My Child?

In light of the current vaccine controversy, the goal of this guide was to provide you with a well-rounded view on vaccinations. Because most of us were raised with the mainstream pro-vaccine point of view, I feel it is important to be become knowledgeable about both sides of the story. This book is not an anti-vaccine treatise; even though I chose to not vaccinate my own sons, I embrace all points of view and encourage, most of all, an informed health choice, and accommodate vaccinating families with separated thimerosal-free shots in my office.

Many parents come to my office and vaccine safety workshops in search of an easy answer to the complex question about what to do regarding childhood vaccinations. Unlike our parents and grandparents, we live in a well-informed age, where the doctor's opinion is not always treated as the absolute. As a result, we question our physicians on everything from choice of medicine to vaccinations. There is not one simple method that works for each family. You will need to find the correct way that suits your child's needs and works within your view of health—which can expand and grow as you take the path of parenthood. Living in the twenty-first century allows us to reap the benefits from standard medicine as well as time-honored natural approach traditions that have been successfully used for centuries.

In weighing the benefits versus risks of the illnesses and vaccines, you will come to the right decision for your child, whether it be to give all the recommended shots, selective vaccination, or none at all. The confusion for many lies in the fact that our children suffer less from common infectious illnesses, in part due to immunizations. On the other hand, children are considered less healthy than in the past while suffering with more chronic diseases and unusual conditions such as ADHD, hyperactivity, delays, and chronic allergies that some have linked to the shots.

Also, for all of these common childhood diseases, remember that there are easy steps you can take to prevent infection and natural remedies available to treat them should your child succumb. If you are interested in learning more about homeopathic and other natural treatments for these illnesses, please see my book *Natural Baby and Childcare*.

There is not one correct approach. Throughout most of the United States parents currently have the legal right to waive all or some of the shots—though having a choice about your children's healthcare may be threatened in the future. With more immunizations in the research pipelines and computerized vaccine tracking systems being planned, there is concern that we will become more strictly monitored and our privacy invaded. The definitions for allowance of exemptions, especially religious ones, may also be challenged.

If you decide to vaccinate, use the safe shot strategy to minimize, if not prevent, vaccine side effects. As your child grows, your approach may also change—be flexible and always consider the individual needs of your child.

The following is a selected list where you can find more information about vaccinations and holistic health.

www.drfeder.com

DrFeder.com is a resource on homeopathy, holistic medicine, and natural parenting. The website also features a family of experts in the fields of pregnancy, natural childbirth, vaccine safety, naturopathic medicine, nutrition, massage, feng shui, philosophy, and animal health. For your convenience, DrFeder.com also carries a comprehensive line of homeopathic medicines, gemmotherapy, and aromatherapy skin care.

Vaccine Information

Organizations

Centers for Disease Control and Prevention
National Immunization Program
NIP Public Inquiries
Mailstop E-05
1600 Clifton Rd., NE
Atlanta, GA 30333
(800) 232-4636
www.cdc.gov/nip

Health Advocacy in the Public Interest (HAPI)
PO Box 7068
Gunnison, CO 81290
www.hapihealth.com

National Vaccine Information Center (NVIC)
204 Mill St., Suite B1
Vienna, VA 22180
(703) 938-DPT3
www.909shot.com

National Vaccine Injury Compensation Program
Parklawn Building, Room 8A-35
5600 Fishers Lane
Rockville, MD 20857
(800) 338-2382
www.hrsa.gov/osp/vicp

Vaccine Adverse Event Reporting System (VAERS)
P.O. Box 1100
Rockville, MD 20849-1100
(800) 822-7967
www.vaers.hhs.gov

Books and DVDs

What Your Doctor May Not Tell You About Children's Vaccinations by Stephanie Cave M.D., F.A.A.F.P. with Deborah Mitchell (Warner Books, 2001)

"Vaccinations?" DVD by Jay Gordon, M.D., F.A.A.P. (Well-Loved Baby Video Series, Childcare Media, 2007)

The Vaccine Guide: Risks and Benefits for Children and Adults by Randall Neustaedter, OMD (North Atlantic Books, 2002)

Vaccinations: A Thoughtful Parent's Guide: How to Make Safe, Sensible Decisions about the Risks, Benefits, and Alternatives by Aviva Jill Romm (Healing Arts Press, 2001)

Holistic Health

Organizations

American Academy of Osteopathy
3500 DePauw Blvd., Suite 1080
Indianapolis, IN 46268
(317) 879-1881
www.academyofosteopathy.org

The American Association of Naturopathic Physicians
4435 Wisconsin Ave NW Suite 403
Washington, DC 20016
(866) 538-2267
www.naturopathic.org

The American Academy of Pediatrics
141 Northwest Point Boulevard
Elk Grove Village, IL 60007-1098
(847) 434-4000
www.aap.org

Holistic Pediatric Association
1275 Fourth Street, #118
Santa Rosa, CA 95404
(707) 237-5312
www.hpakids.org

International Chiropractic Pediatric Association
327 N Middletown Road
Media, PA 19063
(610) 565-2360
www.icpa4kids.org

La Leche League International
P.O. Box 4079
Schaumburg, IL 60168-4079
(847) 519-7730, (800) LALECHE
www.lalecheleague.org

National Center for Homeopathy
801 N. Fairfax Street, Suite 306
Alexandria, VA   22314
(877) 624-0613
www.homeopathic.org

Physicians Committee for Responsible Medicine
5100 Wisconsin Ave., N.W., Ste 400
Washington, DC 20016
(202) 686-2210
www.pcrm.org

Books, Magazines, and Newsletters

Natural Baby and Childcare: Practical Medical Advice and Holistic Wisdom for Raising Healthy Children from Birth to Adolescence by Lauren Feder, M.D. (Healthy Living Books, 2006)

A Drug-Free Approach to Asperger Syndrome and Autism: Homeopathic Care for Exceptional Kids by Judyth Reichenberg-Ullman, N.D., L.C.S.W., Robert Ullman, N.D., Ian Luepker,N.D. (Picnic Point Press, 2005)

Everybody's Guide to Homeopathic Medicines by Stephen Cummings, M.D., and Dana Ullman, M.P.H. (Tarcher, 1997)

Impossible Cure: The Promise of Homeopathy by Amy L. Lansky, Ph.D. (R. L. Ranch Press, 2003)

Homeopathic Self-Care: The Quick & Easy Guide for the Whole Family by Robert Ullman, N.D. and Judyth Reichenberg-Ullman, N.D. (Three Rivers Press, 1997)

How to Raise a Healthy Child in Spite of Your Doctor by Robert S. Mendelsohn, M.D. (Ballantine Books, 1987)

Dr. Mercola's Natural Health Newsletter
www.mercola.com

Mothering Magazine
P.O. Box 1690
Santa Fe, NM 87504
(800)984-8116
www.mothering.com

Ritalin-Free Kids: Safe and Effective Homeopathic Medicine for ADHD and Other Behavioral and Learning Problems by Judyth Reichenberg-Ullman, N.D. M.S.W. and Robert Ullman, N.D. (Three Rivers Press, 2000)

Smart Medicine for Healthier Child: A Practical A-to-Z Reference to Natural and Conventional Treatments for Infants and Children by Janet Zand, N.D., L.Ac., Robert Rountree M.D., and Rachel Walton, M.S.N., C.R.N.P. (Avery, 2004)

definition, 57

occurrence, 58

risks of vaccination, 59–60

symptoms, 57–58

treatment, 59

vaccine, 59

pharmaceutical companies, role of, 36–37

phenol, 33

phosphate buffers, 33

Physicians Committee for Responsible Medicine, 125

Physicians' Desk Reference (PDR), 41

pneumococcal conjugate vaccine (PCV7), 65

pneumococcal polysaccharide vaccine (PPV), 44, 65

pneumococcus, 87–88

  complications, 64–65

  definition, 64

  occurrence, 65

  pneumococcal conjugate vaccine (PCV7), 65

  pneumococcal polysaccharide vaccine (PPV), 65

  Prevnar, 29,65

  risks of vaccination, 66

  symptoms, 64

  vaccine, 65

polio, 19, 31, 32, 33, 34, 35

  complications, 67

definition, 66

inactivated polio virus (IPV), 68, 69

occurrence, 67–68

poliomyelitis, 66

risks of vaccination, 68–69

symptoms, 66–67

vaccine, 68

polyethylene glycol p-isooctylphenyl ether, 33

polymyxin B, 33

polyoxy-ethylene 9-10 nonylphenol, 33

polysorbate 20, 33

polysorbate 80, 34

porcine gelatin, 32

Pozzili, Dr. Paolo, 47

PPD (purified, protein-derivative) test. *See* Mantoux test

Prevnar, 29, 65

"pro-informed-choice" attitude, 5

pro-vaccination viewpoint, 16–28

Q

QuantiFERON TB Gold test (QFT-G), 94

R

reactions, recognizing vaccine, 113–116

Recombivax HB, 46